Contemporary issues in health, medicine, and social policy · *General Editor: John B. McKinlay*

Alternative medicines

Edited by J. Warren Salmon

Alternative medicines

Popular and policy
perspectives

Tavistock Publications · New York · London

First published in 1984 by
Tavistock Publications
in association with Methuen, Inc.
733 Third Avenue, New York,
NY 10017

First published in the U K in 1985 by
Tavistock Publications Ltd
11 New Fetter Lane,
London EC4P 4EE

Printed in the United States of
America

*Library of Congress Cataloging
in Publication Data*
Main entry under title:
Alternative medicines, popular
and policy perspectives.
(Contemporary issues in health,
medicine, and social policy)
Bibliography: p.
Includes index.
1. Therapeutic systems.
2. Therapeutic systems –
Social aspects.
3. Holistic medicine.
I. Salmon, J. Warren.
II. Series.   [DNLM:
1. Holistic Health. W 61 A466]
R733.A48 1984 615.5
84–16218

ISBN 0–422–78700–0
ISBN 0–422–78710–8 (pbk.)

*British Library Cataloguing in
Publication Data*
Alternative medicines. –
(Contemporary issues in health,
medicine, and social policy)
1. Therapeutic systems
I. Salmon, J. Warren   II. Series
615.5   R733

ISBN 0–422–78700–0
ISBN 0–422–78710–8 Pbk

Contents

List of contributors

Editor

J. Warren Salmon PhD is a Professor in the School of Urban Policy and Planning at the University of Illinois at Chicago and Coordinator of the Health Specialization. He has held faculty appointments in the Department of Community Medicine and Environmental Health at Hahnemann University and in the College of Allied Health Sciences at Thomas Jefferson University, both in Philadelphia. His doctorate in Medical Care Organization and Administration is from Cornell University. He has held several administrative, planning, and consulting positions in the health field and written extensively on health policy, corporate involvement in medical care, and the self-care and holistic health movements. He is a contributor to *Issues in the Political Economy of Health Care* in this Contemporary Issues in Health, Medicine, and Social Policy Series.

Contributors

Daniel J. Benor MD is a psychiatrist at the Delaware Valley Mental Health Foundation in Doylestown, Pennsylvania and is on the faculty of Hahnemann University Hospital in Philadelphia. At both he specializes in family therapy. He has a very eclectic, holistic approach to psychiatry and is seeking ways to integrate psychic healing into his practice. He has been lecturing on parapsychology and healing for more than ten years in Israel and the US, and is interested especially in research in healing. He has written a comprehensive review on this subject, soon to be published under the title, *The Psi of Relief.*

Howard S. Berliner is Associate Research Scientist at the Conservation of Human Resources program at Columbia University and Visiting Scholar with the Division of Urban Planning at Columbia. He holds a doctorate in health care organization from Johns Hopkins University. He has held several academic and administrative positions in the health field and has published widely on the development of the American health care system and other issues.

Ronald L. Caplan PhD is an Assistant Professor of Economics at Drew University in Madison, New Jersey. He holds both a masters and doctorate in economics from the University of Massachusetts at Amherst. His dissertation is on the changing nature of self-care in American medical care. Other, more recent, areas of research include the commodification of health care, alternatives in birth and the economics of hospitals.

Effie Poy Yew Chow PhD, RN, CA President, East West Academy of Healing Arts, San Francisco, CA, is a private practitioner and consultant for wellness and optimal personal and organizational performance. She is a specialist in sports and industrial injuries, stress and pain rehabilitation, human sexuality and in the field of aging. She developed the Integrated Healing System (IHS) using East/West theories and practices now in research at the Columbia Lutheran Home for the Aging in Seattle, WA. She is vice chairperson, Ad Hoc Committee on Hypertension in Minority Populations of the National

Heart, Lung and Blood Institute (NHLBI) of the National Institutes of Health (NIH), the Department of Health and Human Services (DHHS), and was on the National Advisory Council to The Secretary of DHHS on Health Professions' Education. She is an international lecturer and has lectured at over fifty universities in the US. She has received the distinguished award for outstanding contribution to the science of acupuncture in the US.

Harris L. Coulter PhD is a writer and consultant in Washington, DC. His principal work to date has been *Divided Legacy: A History of the Schism in Medical Thought* (3 vols, Wehawken Book Co., 1973, 1975, 1977) which is an investigation of medical ideas. He has also written extensively on homoeopathic medicine. His most recent book is *DPT – A Shot in the Dark?* (co-authored by Barbara Loe Fisher), to be published early in 1985 by Harcourt Brace Jovanovich.

James S. Gordon MD is Clinical Associate Professor in the Departments of Psychiatry and Community and Family Medicine at the Georgetown University School of Medicine in Washington, DC, and a trustee of the American Holistic Medicine Association. For ten years he was a research psychiatrist at the National Institute of Mental Health. He has written two books on alternative mental health services for adolescents and was the author of the Special Study on Alternative Mental Health Services for President Carter's Commission on Mental Health. He is co-editor of *Health for the Whole Person: The Complete Guide to Holistic Medicine* (Bantam, 1981) and *Mind, Body and Health: Toward an Integral Medicine* (Human Sciences Press, 1984), and co-author of *New Directions in Medicine* (Aurora, 1984).

Arthur Kleinman is an anthropologist and psychiatrist who is Professor of Medical Anthropology and Psychiatry at Harvard. He is the editor of *Culture, Medicine and Psychiatry: A Journal of Comparative Cross-Cultural Research*, and of the Culture, Illness and Healing book series (both of which are published by D. Reidel Publishing Company). His research has centered on cultural influence on illness and care. His field research has been in Taiwan, the People's Republic of China, and in the US.

He has co-edited seven books including *The Relevance of Social Science for Medicine* (with Leon Eisenberg) (D. Reidel), *Culture and Depression* (with Byron Good) (in press), and *Normal and Abnormal Behavior in Chinese Culture* (D. Reidel). His book, *Patients and Healers in the Context of Culture* (University of California Press, 1980) has won the Welcome Medal of the Royal Institute of Anthropology of Great Britain and Ireland. Kleinman is a member of the Institute of the National Academy of Sciences.

Rosemary C R Taylor is Associate Professor of Sociology and Director of the Community Health Program at Tufts University, Boston. Her doctorate in sociology was awarded by the University of California, Santa Barbara. She has taught at Harvard University and held fellowships from the National Endowment for the Humanities and the Bunting Institute, Radcliffe College. She is currently writing a book on illness prevention policies and popular attitudes towards health in the US. Her publications include *Coops, Communes and Collectives* (with J. Case), Pantheon, 1979. Recent articles are drawn from research concerning the historical development of social welfare programs and health policy strategies in western Europe.

Introduction

J. Warren Salmon

A specter is haunting scientific medicine: the specter of alternative approaches to health and healing. A popular resurgence of interest and activity has recently manifested in a wide variety of new and age-old therapeutic modalities which challenge the contemporary form of medicine in advanced western societies. This book explores some of their differences and their implications.

From ancient times to the present, the organized activity of healing historically developed in stages. These were intricately related to culture and economy, as well as to objective disease patterns and the local understandings and interpretations of disease etiology. Everyday health practices were supported by socially designated healers, who received instruction in a body of knowledge about health and illness and the use of herbal remedies and other natural forms of treatment. The knowledge passed on from generation to generation of practitioners was often esoteric in nature, requiring long periods of study and practice. Discoveries, and commercial and cultural exchanges, expanded the practical content of various treatments over time.

Distinct medicines arose in different parts of the world.

Today numerous systems of medicine continue to co-exist with western medicine.[1] The traditional medicines that evolved in China, Japan, Tibet, and in the Arab world are pre-eminent in these eastern societies today. The yogic and ayurvedic medicines also have large constituencies even beyond the national borders of India where they originated. Indigeneous medicines, such as found among native Americans and within southern hemisphere cultures still provide shamanistic healing and serve as sources of folk remedies (Frank 1963; Halifax 1979). These may serve populations that lack primary care services of western medicine, or they may be sought out by individuals and families who prefer them for a variety of reasons even though western medicine is available.

Each such system of medicine arose in societies where the level of cultural, social, and economic development was ancient or feudal. Most have been gradually advanced rather haphazardly by their practitioners, often aided by contemporary scientific medical findings. Attempts to upgrade several of the nineteenth century western medical practices have also continued. This has been true especially for homoeopathy, naturopathy, osteopathy, and later chiropractic (Shryock 1936, 1960; Rothstein 1972; Coulter 1973, 1982). The point needs to be made, however, that no competing system has systematically assembled a body of knowledge expressed more fully in texts, refereed journal articles, and clinical studies than scientific medicine.

Scientific medicine as predominant

Scientific medicine has become the term commonly used to define the theoretical framework and medical procedures of western society, which have become officially sanctioned by the organized medical profession. In the later years of last century, scientific medicine emerged in Europe and America as an advance beyond allopathy as the germ theory provided an explanation and later treatments for various infectious diseases. In contrast to homoeopathy, allopathy combated disease through remedies and procedures producing effects different from the signs and symptoms produced by the treated disease. The Flexner Report of 1910 provoked the reorganization of medical education in the US and extended the latter upgraded form of medicine into the entirety of health care delivery (Berliner 1975). Financial support by the Rockefeller and Carnegie foundations for scientific medicine came in its wake (Brown 1979). American and European political, economic, and cultural hegemony across the twentieth century has assured its dominance over other systems of medicine throughout the world.

This subsequent dominance of scientific medicine was assumed through its theoretical exposition, clinical elaboration, and technological advancement. By focusing systematically on the biological aspects of human disease, this particular system of medicine has continued with an ever-sharpening focus on anatomy, physiology, biochemistry, microbiology, molecular biology, surgery, pharmacology, genetics, and its other subject matter. Its clinical activity has branched in numerous specialties and sub-specialties over the last seventy-five years (Stevens 1971). The frontiers of "science" in medicine continually promise greater discoveries to shed new understanding on the physical nature and treatment of diseases in our current civilization.

However, there is much more to the picture. Anthropologists examining previous historical periods have clearly demonstrated healing's earlier interstices with culture and economy. Yet, the form and content of scientific medicine has been widely interpreted to be independent of the social context in which it has developed and presently reigns. It is inherently assumed to have an internally coherent, self-evident, and objective validity. This assumed validity furthermore is so taken for granted in western society that suggestions that other systems of medicine may also have validity are often rejected out of hand. Western superiority in economic, technological, and military spheres has perpetuated the assumption that scientific medicine is likewise far superior to its predecessors and competitors. Even the referent of "scientific" exemplifies having reached a pinnacle of achievement, implying that other systems of medicine are non-scientific, being based upon lesser foundations. As a consequence, the predominant thinking about scientific medicine neglects consideration of what usually is applied to alternative systems – to examine the rootedness and history of its conceptions and systems of thought, contrasting them to competing systems. As is the tendency in all social institutions in modern society, medicine has become reified, often viewed in a crystalized form.

Taken out of its historical context of continual development and change, scientific medicine has been given a life of its own apart from the human actions and the power of the vested social interests that create and maintain it. In this regard, the specific ideological and institutional functions that this kind of medicine performs in modern capitalist society have become reflected in its practice (McKinlay 1984). Medicine contributes substantially to the accumulation of corporate profit. Besides pharmaceuticals, hospital equipment and supplies, construction, investment banking, and other associated industries, the for-profit delivery of services in the "new medical industrial complex" marks one of the most lucrative investment areas in the American economy (Ehrenreich and Ehrenreich 1970; Goddard 1973; Relman 1980; Salmon 1984). In addition, institutionalized medicine serves to rationalize and legitimate the existing social order (Waitzkin and Waterman 1974; Navarro 1976; Waitzkin 1978, 1983). Medicalization of the society has provoked extensive ethical, moral, and legal commentary (Zola 1972, 1975; Illich 1976), and the content of medicine, let alone its social organization, has historically been inseparable from racist and sexist tendencies, along with performing other social control functions (Ehrenreich and English 1978).

The paradigmatic critique

Notwithstanding its vast accomplishments in disease eradication, scientific medicine has drawn significant criticism of late, going well beyond problems of its costs and organization. The disarray in the delivery of services and its escalating costs have fueled an increasing scrutiny over medicine's content. The paradigm of scientific medicine, its basic assumptions about health and disease, and its practical approach to the patient have each come under considerable attack (Frankl 1965; Illich 1976; Carlson 1975a, 1975b). Moreover, the iatrogenic quality of technological medicine has been focused on besides its ineffectiveness in addressing certain aspects of chronic degenerative illnesses (Cochrane 1972; Office of Technology Assessment 1978; Kane 1980).

Kuhn's *The Structure of Scientific Revolutions* (1962) had a tremendous influence on thinking in the natural and social sciences. Using physics as an example, Kuhn simply described how scientific ideas were generated; how they took hold in the community of researchers; how they were refined and expanded; and how and why they were eventually replaced. According to Kuhn, imperfections in paradigms always leave certain unanswered questions and generate efforts by researchers to make the evidence fit the theory. Adherents to the old paradigms and those claiming the relative merits of new proposed ones clash.

It is not at all clear that medicine should be critiqued along the line of Kuhn's reasoning for the physical sciences. In the 1940s Henry Sigerist argued that medicine is not so much a natural as a social science (Marti-Ibanez 1960). Despite medical scientists maintaining a different stance, the perspectives of public health, epidemiology, demography, sociology, social psychology, and social anthropology give substantial support to Sigerist's view. The fact remains that while healing is undeniably a social process, scientific medicine has generally downplayed the interconnections of its social aspects to the practical content of therapeutics.

Nevertheless, Kuhn's work fashioned the arguments of social critics of established medicine, who were quick to point out anomalies in its paradigmatic structure. In actuality, the conceptual framework utilized by modern medicine is highly complex and contains many paradigms. This furthur complicates attempts to understand modern medicine as a social institution. The paradox remains that as the content of medicine becomes increasingly refined, the social dynamics of health care delivery and its implications to the individual become more complicated and more difficult to delineate.

Thus, the calls for a "new medicine," or more properly, a new orientation to healing, have been resounded by practitioners of a variety of alternative therapeutic modalities (Brown 1974; Pelletier 1976, 1979; Krippner and Villoldo 1976; Meek 1977; Fosshage and Olsen 1978; Joy 1979; Otto and Knight 1979; Albright and Albright 1980; Dossey 1983). From within nursing, advocates hope their colleagues will utilize the new orientation in their development of an expanded professional role (Flynn 1980a, 1980b; Rogers 1980; Blattner 1981; Krieger 1981). This developing critique of scientific medicine, and the expanded or opposing thought about health and healing, have been substantially influenced by examinations of alternative systems of medicine.

Criticisms have not been confined to those outside the medical profession (Menninger 1976; Engel 1977; Lambert 1978; Mendelsohn 1979; Sobel 1979; Hastings, Fadiman, and Gordon 1980). Physicians over the years have been implying the need for a broader understanding of illness and an expanded terrain for both treatment and prevention of the individual's disease in social medicine, public health, community medicine, occupational and environmental medicine, social psychiatry, psychosomatics, family medicine, and humanistic medicine. Predictably, the collective impact of these currents within the house of scientific medicine can be said to be negligible to date. Representatives of the medical profession and the institutions it controls may no longer be able to maintain an immutability toward these identified problems in the face of stronger progressive struggles and government and corporate strategies for reform.

More recently, there is promise, and evidence, of change towards alternative therapeutics by the medical profession, though some quarters still are resolute in their resistance to the wave of new practitioners and their insufficiently studied remedies (Callan 1979; Relman 1979; "Orthodox Medicine" 1979). Previously, physicians in general would not tolerate, let alone associate with, non-licensed practitioners, other physicians who practiced unsanctioned therapies, or chiropractors. In the US legal actions brought by the chiropractic organizations have made the official stance more congruent with the actual behavior of a growing minority of doctors who refer to practitioners of alternative therapies. The fact remains that patients in the US and throughout Europe are utilizing chiropractors, acupuncturists, psychic and spiritual healers, homoeopaths, naturopaths, and many more holistic-styled practitioners, and increasingly telling their physicians about the benefits derived. In Britain, perhaps a greater openness is found among younger physicians who report a positive attitude toward practitioners who used to be labeled deviant or even quacks (Reilly 1983). As alternative systems of medicine are publicized more widely to regular physician, nursing, and allied health audiences, larger numbers will continue to seek to broaden their scope of practice, display a willingness to interact with other practitioners, and carry on experimentation toward integration with their trained practices.

Two related and intertwined social developments have contributed to the intellectual and practical search into the realm of alternative systems of medicine. The first concerns the broader rhythm for health in American and European societies. This quest for health has provoked reconceptualizations of health, healing, and human existence. The second stems from the organizational and financing problems in dominant health care institutions. Their pending restructuring over the next few decades presents varied opportunities to advocates of alternative approaches to health and healing.

The social concerns for a broader health

A confluence of economic, social, and cultural factors account for the upsurge of interest in health by Americans and Britons, and Europeans (Argument-Sonderband 1983). These come from within the ranks of workers demanding safe jobs; from environmentalists and opponents to nuclear energy; from the women's movement through Counter-Culture and New Age activities. Peace movement groups, such as the Physicians For Social Responsibility in the US, have identified the increasing danger of nuclear conflict as the penultimate public health issue.

Not just limited to these social struggles, maintaining and enhancing one's health has become a primary pursuit of people involved in nutrition, fitness, "lifestyle" adjustments, and a variety of spiritual practices, such as yoga and meditation. Many of these activities have been fueled by narcissistic societal tendencies (Lasch 1978) and spurred on by media hoopla on the nascent trendiness of self-care (Salmon and Berliner 1982).

The bulk of the rising social concerns for health and its varied pursuits are generally tangential to mainstream medical theory and practice. Critics have charged that the paradigmatic structure of scientific medicine does not readily allow for health defined in a broader sense. This may be the main cause of popular disaffection toward the particular form of medicine associated with conventional health care.

Last decade's resurgence of the holistic health movement in Western Europe and the United States can also be attributed to the increasing dissatisfaction with the present systems of health care delivery (Berliner and Salmon 1980). A recent writer in the *British Medical Journal* described alternative therapeutics as one of the few growth industries in contemporary Britain (Smith 1983). Defining this "movement" is problematic beyond grouping together all practitioners who place themselves against or outside of conventional medicine (Berkeley Holistic Health Center 1978; Kaslof 1978; LaPatra 1978; Cousins 1979). Advocates of holistic health assert as a cardinal principle the notion of the fundamental and integral unity of the body, the mind, and the spirit. Included in this notion of health is not merely the presence of somatic (physical) signs and symptoms, but also the state of the relation of the mind with the body's functioning, and the person's sense of connection to the spiritual realm. A grab-bag of specific therapeutic interventions have been called "holistic," even while they may not address all three aspects of the "whole" person in either theory or practice. The growing popularity of these concepts and therapies has surely ushered in a renewed openness toward nineteenth century western medical practices, as well as toward oriental medicines and several of the traditional and indigenous therapeutic systems which are still prevalent across the globe.

Difficulties arise in attempting to combine the various competing *systems* to conventional medicine due to their diverse philosophical, social, and cultural backgrounds. For one thing, there are substantial variations in their degree of documented validation and explanation. Nevertheless, the general point that can be made about alternative systems, is that most contain concepts of health and illness that go beyond the crude materialism of scientific medicine. Disease, according to scientific medicine, is a disordered biological state, described in terms of physical science and treated generally independently from social behavior and intrapsychic processes, let alone larger cosmological forces. When given attention, such factors are too often isolated under the rubric of psychological problems and referred out to a separate practitioner who is usually not involved with the physical aspects of the problem. While in modern medical practice today this deficiency is being increasingly addressed, theoretical unity of mental, emotional, and spiritual aspects of healing with the somatic has yet to be achieved.

Recent thinking about health has been greatly influenced by existentialist, humanistic, and transpersonal thought as well as by modern explorers of the age-old traditions of Zen and Tibetan Buddhism, Sufism, Hinduism, and mystical Judaism (Frankl 1955; Needleman and Lewis 1976). As modern psychological theory has been transformed by these intellectual currents, the concepts of health and healing have changed as well. These broader metaphysical understandings seem to require and strengthen a more human connection between practitioner and patient in the healing encounter. In contrast to scientific medicine, most alternatives share a notion of "energy" which accounts for biochemical and physiological systems, but also may include more subtle aspects of a human "electromagnetic field." The Chinese have referred to it as "chi," and the Japanese in shiatsu and akido call it "ki." Yogis have labeled it "prana." There have also been western definitions: Hippocrates' "physics;" "archeus" by Paracelsus; Samuel Hahnemann spoke of the "vital force." (White and Krippner (1977) catalog four and a half pages of such terms from sources around the world through five millennia of recorded history.) While slightly different, each presupposes an innate healing potential within the person that at times may be affected by external forces. Those seeking a new medicine refashioned around this notion of a universal healing power usually assign a mystical character to their inspirational interventions, along with a call to faith in a higher order. These are not all medieval conceptions either, for practitioners are attempting to suitably update this orientation for today's practice.

Perhaps within the broader rhythm for health in modern societies is some rebellion against the rationalization we face in all spheres of social and cultural activity, and against the penetrating effect of reification on our consciousness and daily life. The attraction to Alternative medicines with their different conceptions of health, healing, and human existence reflects what might be expected with the apparent breaking down of one system and its organization as it may be giving way to another.

The crisis in health care delivery

Over the last fifteen years, both the United States and United Kingdom have witnessed an exponential rise in medical care costs. Health care expenditures now represent a significantly higher proportion of Gross National Product, and of government expenses than they ever have. The reduction of this cost inflation has become the central focus of health policy in both the Reagan and Thatcher administrations. Each has attempted to substantially reduce their respective governments' health care outlays. This may prove to have severe health consequences for certain population groups. While policy-makers mainly seek contraction of health care provider revenues and curtailment of inappropriate and excessive utilization, consumers are being forced to bear a greater share of costs. This neo-conservative premise assumes a more prudent use of the health care system. Indirectly, it may increase competition from alternative medical services, as patients may likely use these to lower their out-of-pocket expenditures.

Amid policies of cost containment, cutbacks, and higher consumer co-payments, the maldistribution of health care services in the US, and the regional allocations for Britain's National Health Service, remain important political issues. Neither system of care adequately concerns itself with the distribution of disease in each population, nor are high priorities placed upon addressing social etiologies of disease in either society (Eyer and Sterling 1977; Turshen 1977; Sidel and Sidel 1979). Meanwhile, public dissatisfaction grows with the increasing cost burden, the perceived impersonality of care, and the alienation found within bureaucratic provider settings. People are increasingly coming to consider that the problems and limitations of conventional health care are not exclusively confined to the organization of each country's delivery system.

Health policy analysts maintain that the cost crisis is intricately related to the effectiveness of specific services comprising the practice of scientific medicine. McKeown (1971) and Powles (1973) found that the interventions of medicine were not the primary reason behind declines in mortality until the mid-twentieth century. Rather, public health measures and rising standards of living accounted more for the improvements in health. From analyses of more recent data,

McKinlay and McKinlay (1977, 1979) urge that social and environmental factors be granted greater attention in order to reduce the major causes of disease and disability today. Policy analysts of opposing political perspectives now see increased investment in technological medicine bringing limited returns in improved health relative to its costs. Given these limitations of modern medicine and the demonstrated ineffectiveness of numerous medical procedures, there is ample justification for a reappraisal of the significance and wisdom of expanding scientific medicine (McKinlay 1981). In concert with such a reappraisal, a worthwhile review of the philosophical and practical contributions of alternative systems of medicine, and the new thinking influenced by them, is in order.

The chapters of the volume 'Alternative medicines: popular and policy perspectives'

This book recognizes the genuine interest that has risen in the many traditional practices and nineteenth century medicines on the part of conventional health care practitioners, as well as the public. With the increasing attention to this collection of diverse theories and practices in occidental societies, there is a need for a more informed public that recognizes some of the implications and potential benefits from the utilization of alternative therapeutics. The book is intended to provide a better understanding of selected unorthodox systems and to offer a variety of viewpoints on their public acceptance and related policy issues. This should help foster a more thorough consideration of ways that alternative systems of medicine can advance the nature and practice of healing in the modern western world. At such time when aspects of alternatives are more integrated into conventional health care delivery, their complementary, adjunctive, or substitutive role will be better understood. The following chapters have been prepared to identify selected issues and to provide a sketch of popular and policy perspectives.

Scientific medicine since Flexner

The tremendous success of biomedical practice in the last fifty years must be acknowledged. Nevertheless, Howard S. Berliner believes that the limitations of scientific medicine must be fully understood in order not to reproduce them in the superseding forms of medicine. His perspective is concerned with how medical knowledge has historically been organized and controlled, noting the intersections of ideology, culture, and economy with medicine. His past examinations have viewed alterations in the content and organization of medicine as the political economy of health care has moved toward greater concentration and centralization in the economy (Berliner 1975, 1977, 1983; Berliner and Salmon 1980). Dr Berliner here maintains that alternatives challenge both the organization and content of scientific medicine in most crucial ways. He examines several factors which have provoked popular discontent with modern medical care, including: changes in disease distribution; demographic changes in the population structure; alterations in the patient–physician relationship; the limitations of hospital care; problems with technology and machine-model orientation of modern medicine; the dominance of cure over prevention; and lastly, the mounting costs of medical care. While granting that alternatives may pose some rigorous questions, his research has shown that dominant scientific medicine is well entrenched and unlikely to be changed easily. He begins this volume by highlighting the social context of health care within which alternative systems are re-emerging. This analytical focus raises a series of issues that proponents of alternative systems of medicine often overlook when considering extension of their respective medical theories.

Homoeopathy

Homoeopathy represents a western system of medicine that holds significant popularity around the globe, especially outside the US. It was developed by Samuel Hahnemann, a German physician and reformer who died in 1843. In contrast to the heroic practices of allopathy back then (bleeding, purging, leeching, and the use of heavy metals for medication), Hahnemann proposed a more gentle means of aiding the person's resistance to disease. Homoeopathic practice consists of administering a carefully selected, single remedy in infinitely small dosages to stimulate the body's natural defenses.

Currently, a resurgence of interest has begun in America where it previously was a major competing sect to scientific medicine. When the latter was aided by Rockefeller and Carnegie philanthropic support at the turn of the century, homoeopathy's popular and political bases were undermined. In England, homoeopathy has maintained a strong following, which includes among its advocates the Royal family.

Dr Harris Coulter, an authority on its history, details in his chapter how the principles of homoeopathy clearly distinguish its theory and practice from that of scientific medicine. He notes that the empirical approach of homoeopathic provings in practice has been fraught with methodological pitfalls. Yet, he believes that homoeopathy's approach makes for a vastly superior medicine because it recognizes the uniqueness of each individual patient. The primary concern of the homeopathic method is patient "idiosyncrasy." It begins with a structuring of the practitioner–patient relationship toward the acquisition and use of an elaborate history. This concern for the individual patient yields a marked degree of intimacy, responding to a factor the public has complained is absent in conventional medical practice. Dr Coulter closes his chapter by calling for removal of scientific medicine's condemnation and ostracism of homeopathy. For health policy consideration, he recommends separate licensing boards in the United States and other conditions to allow homeopathic practice to be judged in a freer atmosphere.

Chiropractic

Since its American origins around the turn of the century, chiropractic has enjoyed an exceptional existence in the US health care system. Medical sociologists have usually confined chiropractors to a category of "quasi- or deviant practitioners" due to their maligned status by the medical profession. Chiropractors are the chief alternative practitioners who are state-sanctioned with licensing, even though their services have yet to be incorporated into the conventional hospital-based system of care (Manber 1978). On both scientific and economic grounds, the medical profession has vigorously opposed the theory and practice of chiropractic. Nevertheless, it remains the major and most popular "hands-on" body therapy, whose theoretical underpinnings and practice have been borrowed from, and are somewhat supported by, a variety of holistic-styled approaches.

In his chapter, Ronald Lee Caplan reviews how chiropractic has constantly fought for its turf within the US health care system. He notes that its therapeutic interventions are among the few from alternative systems which are reimbursed by the third-party insurance system. (During the last decade chiropractic was granted partial public payment from Medicare and most Medicaid programs.) Dr Caplan examines the development of chiropractic and the differences in its approach from scientific medicine. While he sees the need for more substantial research on spinal manipulation and other aspects of chiropractic, he notes difficulties in advancing this, given the substantial portion of the medical profession which resents the economic competition. Dr Caplan discusses issues related to the need for cooperation among health care professionals of different orientations and skills. He concludes by delineating several hopeful signs within and without chiropractic, noting that popular acceptance of this alternative assures its continued growth and greater influence.

Traditional Chinese medicine

Americans were introduced to the theory, techniques, and accomplishments of Chinese medicine following President Richard Nixon's opening of diplomatic relations with the People's Republic of China in the mid-1970s. However, its philosophical and theoretical bases have not been accorded as much attention as the glamour of specific techniques which have attracted medical practitioners. Today, acupuncture is widely practiced in the US, being granted state licensing for certified professionals in several states. Aspects of one system of medicine, as well as the health care delivery system, are never readily transplanted into a foreign setting without significant alteration (Sidel and Sidel 1972; Lampton 1974, 1977; Kleinman *et al.* 1975; Garfield and Salmon 1981). There is much more to Chinese medicine than the mechanistic applications of acupuncture and herbs or their media presentations. A fuller understanding of the overall system of Chinese medicine and its methodology may aid appreciation of the several age-old systems originating in the East.

In her chapter, Effie Poy Chow summarizes the constructs of Chinese traditional medicine which have evolved from classical times. She delineates several clinical aspects in the diagnosis and treatment of disease, utilizing her observations from the People's Republic of China and her personal practice. Dr Chow reviews the state of this form of medicine in the United States and concludes with a discussion of related policy implications from Chinese medical techniques. She identifies issues pertinent to the rise of other alternative therapeutics that can be learned from the implementation of acupuncture. Her concluding insights offer suggestions for both mainstream medical and alternative practitioners.

Indigenous systems of healing

To borrow a phrase from Mao Zedong, indigenous and traditional medicines from across the globe contain a "great treasure house." As anthropological and medical investigators have shown (Kleinman *et al.* 1975; Ortiz de Montellano 1975; Leslie 1976), many of the indigenous practices are empirically derived. As such, these therapeutic interventions more often than not work in some way to the satisfaction of both practitioners and patients. This has not been as precise and elaborate in most cases as the clinical trials of scientific medicine (though flaws exist in this methodology too) (Chalmers 1981). Alternative systems are usually construed in a negative light by scientific medical observers who criticize inconsistencies with scientific findings and metaphysical notions in their theories, which are at variance to those of scientific medicine. In addition, much of the alternative systems literature has not been suitably updated from classical texts. It is important to recognize that transplanted versions of many indigenous practices are not the best standards for judging the efficacy of such practices nor assessing the merits of the systems. Critics might also note that diligent alternative practitioners in their native nations have recently expanded their knowledge base and upgraded numerous techniques. On the other hand, advocates of indigenous and traditional medicines commonly idolize their practice sometimes beyond the most accurate portrayal of its strengths and limitations.

Drawing upon his extensive investigations of indigenous systems of healing, Arthur Kleinman makes mention of how professional health care in the east is now practiced quite differently from the classical ideology of the traditional profession. In fact, he and others have found that there are numerous "borrowings and adoptions from Western biomedicine." In his chapter, Dr Kleinman discusses the three major arenas of care that constitute any local health care system: popular, folk, and professional. He notes that indigenous practices have not withered and died in societies where western biomedicine has been introduced, but are indeed currently undergoing a revival, particularly in North America and Western Europe. He questions the commercial tendencies in the popular and professional arenas (i.e. in America the holistic health movement and profit-based hospitals in conventional care), feeling that both may further weaken lay care initiatives. He believes that the latter lay activities have over time upheld individuals, families, and their social networks, forming the base of health maintenance. Dr Kleinman categorizes folk healing into both sacred and secular, and modern and traditional. Following a review of literature on the efficacy of several of these practices, he tentatively suggests that they may be effective in healing illness experience, but less so in treating disease. He explores what has been, and can be, learned from indigenous healers in a quite positive light. Dr Kleinman further delineates clinically relevant categories for comparing folk with other therapeutic relationships – criteria that can be utilized to evaluate and learn from indigenous and traditional medicines. The application of such comparisons may open up greater appreciation for their contributions to people's health. In his conclusion, Dr Kleinman shares thoughts regarding the changing boundaries in relationships between the three arenas of care. He notes that popular and other indigenous healing is challenging the professional sector for greater control over health resources, decisions, and practices. This dynamic holds significant implications for health care.

Psychic healing

Spectacular advances may be on the horizon of technological medicine (Thomas 1983a, 1983b); however, there is reason to believe that financial access to them by the entire population will be severely limited (Mechanic 1979; Evans 1983). Corporate purchaser groups and government planners foresee rationing health services according to ability to pay (Goldbeck 1978). Rising medical costs either crimp the former's profit margins, or add to the latter's federal deficit (Salmon 1977, 1978, 1982). Given the likelihood that larger numbers of people may be denied certain costly procedures and service in coming years, there is an urgent social need to explore cheaper, more effective modalities of care, ones that can be popularly based under the control of families and communities. In past times, such alternatives have gained favor during periods of economic decline and restricted access to the medical profession.

Today, a sizeable number of Americans, Britons, and Europeans, even with the means to obtain regular medical services, are choosing alternatives, particularly those consigned to the category of mind therapies. These choices are for supplements to, and sometimes substitutes for, their conventional medical care. These preferences for non-technological healing are in part promoted by the social currents running through the women's health movement, as well as Counter-Culture and New Age followings. Playing an important part are the spiritual groups from the fundamentalist Christian movement through the varieties of eastern religious infusions (Zaretsky 1972; Cox 1979). The media has surely fostered attention on novelty human experiences brought from the margins of society, further promulgating psychic and spiritual healing and other parapsychological phenomena in the public mind. A plethora of books, news reports, and popular television shows have helped to revive a long history of American and British interest in the esoteric and occult. More people now are aware of psychic healing as an option for dealing with several kinds of physical and emotional problems. This modality (and variations on its theme in a wide variety of mind–body therapies) has been gaining greater legitimacy through efforts of serious investigators and medical practitioners (Grad 1971–72; Ehrenwald 1977; Harman 1981). Psychic healing and its derivatives offer an attractive alternative, both in being a safe, non-invasive therapy and in its potential cost-effectiveness for certain illnesses and certain patients.

In his chapter, Daniel Benor reviews evidence supporting the effectiveness of psychic healing as a therapeutic modality. He speaks to the existence of bio-energies functioning in nature that are largely ignored and insufficiently explored by conventional science. While recognizing that no clear theory exists to substantiate, or even adequately describe, intentional interpersonal healing, he describes some experiments and activities in healing and their relation to parapsychology and other new areas of scientific research. This may lead to a more scientific understanding of healing, though still necessitating more research with a new framework to recognize unseen phenomena through more creative and rigorous protocols. He regards the attempts for broadening paradigms in medicine and the physical sciences as leading to a greater explanatory and predictive basis to healing. Dr Benor argues that other dimensions of reality may be entered into by the healer and healee during episodes of psychic healing. He mentions that select individuals with demonstrated healing abilities at certain times seem to have a latent sense for an altered connection to time, space, and matter. These healers experience reality at a different level of perception beyond the basic five senses and maintain they possess an inner power derived from universal sources. Explorations in consciousness expansion in certain scientific circles are already contributing much to the advance of healing (White 1974; Harman 1981). From his studies, Dr Benor has come to respect the energy of order, intelligence, and compassion found in many healers, believing psychic healing offers practical suggestions for improving effectiveness of therapeutic interventions by all health care practitioners.

Alternative medicine and the medical encounter

Assessments of the exact reasons for the emergence and revival of Alternative medicines and therapeutics have been varied. Proponents and enthusiasts of specific orientations and modalities can only be partially relied upon, as can also be the detractors of alternatives. One major problem faced by the remaining commentators attempting to examine the broader social interest in health and healing has been definitional problems of what constitutes unorthodox or Alternative medicines and practices in addition to lay initiatives and self-care. There are wide variations here. Lack of substantial empirical backup accounts for emphases given to certain aspects of the overall social dimensions to the whats and whys of people's explorations of various health practices. The British Holistic Medical Association plans to investigate what alternative therapies are being used and why people believe they work (Lister 1983). For sure, the surrounding social dynamics are complex, and a firmer data base awaits its assembling on the nature and extent of the use of alternatives; the knowledge of and attitudes toward them; and the social characteristics of people who utilize them. Equally important are more thorough analyses of relevant health policy issues. Some preliminary work has begun to at least comment on the implications of alternative practices in health planning, certification and licensure of practitioners, assessments of therapeutic effacacy, federal/state funding, and public and private health insurance reimbursement (Carlson 1975a; Ardell 1976; Fink 1976; Salmon and Berliner 1980a/b).

In her chapter, Rosemary Taylor explores some of the social dimensions to the flourishing interest in alternative forms of healing. She provides evidence of the growth in numbers of alternative practitioners in the US and Britain. By reviewing various authors' assessments on the rise of alternatives, her critical essay differentiates these forms from scientific medicine. Dr Taylor's major thrust is to ascertain related societal, cultural, and health system factors. She notes the class-based followings of previous and present alternative practices. She notes that different alternatives seem to have divergent appeals to different audiences. However, Dr Taylor places most emphasis on the changing nature of the modern medical encounter for the current expressed dissatisfaction. She believes that a fall in public regard for medical doctors, not disenchantment with medical science, has more to do with the turn toward alternative therapeutics. Consumerist tendencies over recent years make the patient–practitioner relationship anachronistic. Choosing alternatives and self-care may represent a reaction to contemporary medicine's increasing jurisdiction over social life.

Holistic health centers in the United States

As Illich (1976) and others suggest (Cousins 1976, 1983), perhaps the bureaucratic and technological context that enshrines modern medical encounters accounts for some of the lack of healing, and even inflicts certain damage on patients. Iatrogenesis in established health care institutions may partially result from the form, characteristics, and power relations of their organization. In his classic study of shamanistic healing, Frank (1963) examined how its social context carried symbolic meaning from cultural and religious influences on everyday life. In this primitive situation, illness was viewed as a community affair; the relationship between practitioner and patient was quite intimate; and natural, spiritual, and cosmological forces were usually invoked. Often, healing of the family and tribe was ritualized in order to mobilize community attention to the member who was ill. In western society, attention to the social context of patient illness and the immediate environment for healing is beginning to emerge within holistic health circles. The generally staid, bureaucratic hospital is increasingly viewed, even by conventional health care professionals, as in need of significant change to humanize its patient services, in addition to providing better working conditions. Prospects for more creative organizational development, and the integration of various alternative modalities with conventional medicine, appear to be greater in newly styled centers that are blossoming across the US and Western Europe (Hastings, Fadiman, and Gordon 1980).

In his chapter, James Gordon details the growth of these multidisciplinary therapeutic and educational organizations in the US. As with the free clinic movement and women's health centers, he sees holistic health centers responding to popular requests for alternative settings of care, as well as alternative therapeutics *and* new practitioner–patient relationships for care. From his associations with and study of several centers, he lays out how the concepts of holism are embodied in their practices. He lists some of their salient organizational characteristics and discusses how he sees the practice of regular scientific medicine being influenced by these initial models. Dr Gordon is hopeful about influences from the holistic health movement on mainstream medical care. He mentions several types of therapies and modalities, providing examples of their implementation in various centers. His concluding comments are pertinent to where the practice of Alternative medicines and holistic health care should proceed over the next decade. He offers sage advice to alternative practitioners who wish to advance their efforts and increase their public acceptance.

Defining health and reorganizing medicine

The goal of medicine as a social institution is to further, or to accomplish, the healing of societal members who are sick, as well as prevent their getting sick in the first place. Central to an examination of the practical content of any system of medicine then should be its effectiveness in reducing the disease burden within the treated population over time. Toward this end, extensive explanatory capabilities regarding health and illness, in addition to disease, are required (in other words, the nature and content of its theories and principles and its assumptions about the human being within the context of larger social life). Also required for its practice is an armamentarium of interventions with empirically-derived effacacy. However, proper diagnosis and treatment entails much more than the clinical picture of the individual patient.

Medicine must be correctly construed as a social science (Sigerist 1960). The locus of medical practice – even granting exclusive focus on disease – must extend not only beyond the organ, but also beyond the organism (Wartofsky 1975). Wartofsky sees the appropriate human ontology, or construction of reality, to be a socio-historical and cultural system of individuals, articulated by their concrete and specific forms of life activities in society. Thus, the "science" of medicine, embedded in the social institution of medicine, takes on social, political, and cultural characteristics that shape its principles just as they shape its practice. Given increasing social conflicts over the origins of disease in modern society (Totman 1979; Eyer 1984), the corporate class in the US has been taking steps to gain more strategic control over the "health" of its workforce (Salmon 1978). Corporate and government efforts to reorganize the respective health care systems in the US and UK have a strong bearing upon prospects for a new "health-oriented" medicine that may emerge from syntheses of scientific and various alternative systems of medicine and new adjunctive therapeutics.

In the last chapter of this volume, I review definitions of health offered from sources within the established health care system and what a few of the more holistic writers suggest to expand them. The broader social, ecological, and cosmological parameters to the concept of health are examined. I explore some dimensions of the "paradigm shift" in medicine, relating back to points made previously about the nature of health (Carlson 1975a; Ferguson 1978; Capra 1982). Here I briefly describe implications from the "new physics" and the suggested ways that consciousness is believed to impact health and healing (Capra 1977; Bohm 1980; Dossey 1983). My discussion emphasizes the current institutional context of health care delivery. Quite directly, I attempt to portray that the significance of debates on the definition of health, its generation and restoration, must be viewed in the light of political economic developments. The problems of escalating costs and questionable effectiveness of present health care systems render these deliberations more than a mere intellectual concern. The challenges to the ideological hegemony of scientific medicine may lead greater numbers of people to question not only the nature and content of its current practice, but also the parties who profit from its dominance (Salmon 1984).

In my opinion, the paradigm builders for a "new medicine" are trying in both human and intellectual terms to work their way through to deeper realities that form the basis of inquiry into human existence. This orientation may lead us to examine human possibilities and capabilities assessed in the totality of society and the world, not just measured as individual achievement or, in point here, as individual health. In our effort to create a world where the inner and outer life of all people is dominated more by human, and less by economic, motives and values, we may realize that an indispensable condition for our improved collective health is a changed social order. My conclusion offers brief thoughts regarding the future course of formulating a new epistemology of medicine. Reconceptualizations of health, healing, and human existence that are popularly grounded will be needed. Here I believe examinations of alternative systems of medicine, and the newer, integrated perspectives on health and healing influenced by them, may provide avenues for new formulations.

Note

1 For purposes of this volume, *alternative systems of medicine* are distinguished from the potpourri of modalities usually seen to make up the contents of "holistic health care." The latter has served as a catchall for a diverse and eclectic sampling of therapies and practices, many of which have been extracted from ancient, traditional, and nineteenth century western alternative systems of medicine, besides a variety of newly formulated therapeutic techniques. The point of distinction relies upon a body of theoretical knowledge and a set of therapeutic interventions codified as a system of medicine over time by a socially recognized group of practitioners. While the authors of this volume may at times in their analyses consider the collectivity of alternative therapeutics, the thrust of the book is to present a discussion of selected alternative *systems* to scientific medicine and their theoretical, practical, and policy implications.

References

Albright, P. and Albright, B.P. (eds) (1980) *Body, Mind and Spirit.* Brattleboro, Vermont: The Stephen Greene Press.

Ardell, D.B. (1976) From Omnibus Tinkering to High-Level Wellness: The Movement Toward Holistic Health Planning. *American Journal of Health Planning* 1: 15–34.

Argument-Sonderband (ed.) (1983) *Alternative Medizin.* Berlin: Argument-Verlag.

Berkeley Holistic Health Center (1978) *The Holistic Health Handbook.* Berkeley: And/Or Press.

Berliner, H.S. (1975) A Larger Perspective on the Flexner Report. *International Journal of Health Services* 5: 573–92.

——(1977) *Philanthropic Foundations and Scientific Medicine.* Unpublished dissertation, Johns Hopkins University.

——(1983) Medical Modes of Production. In A. Treacher and P. Wright (eds) *The Social Construction of Medicine.* Edinburgh: University of Edinburgh Press.

Berliner, H.S. and Salmon, J.W. (1980) The Holistic Alternative to Scientific Medicine: History and Analysis. *International Journal of Health Services* 10: 133–47.

Blattner, B. (1981) *Holistic Nursing.* Englewood Cliffs, NJ: Prentice-Hall.

Bohm, D. (1980) *Wholeness and The Implicate Order.* London: Routledge & Kegan Paul.

Brown, B. (1974) *New Mind, New Body*. New York: Harper & Row.

Brown, E.R. (1979) *Rockefeller Medicine Men: Medicine and Capitalism in America*. Berkeley: University of California Press.

Callan, J.P. (1979) Holistic Health or Holistic Hoax. *Journal of the American Medical Association* 241: 1156.

Capra, F. (1977) *The Tao of Physics*. New York: Bantam Books.

——(1982) *The Turning Point: Science, Society, and the Rising Culture*. New York: Bantam Books.

Carlson, R.J. (1975a) *The End of Medicine*. New York: John Wiley.

——(ed.) (1975b) *The Frontiers of Science and Medicine*. Chicago: Henry Regnery.

Chalmers, T.C. (1981) The Clinical Trial. *Milbank Memorial Fund Quarterly Health and Society* 59(3): 324–39.

Cochrane, A. (1972) *Effectiveness and Efficiency*. London: Nuffield Provincial Hospitals Trust.

Coulter, H. (1973) *Homeopathic Influences on Nineteenth Century Allopathic Therapeutics*. Washington, DC: American Institutes of Homoeopathy.

——(1982) *Divided Legacy: A History of the Schism in Medical Thought* (vol. 3). Washington, DC: McGrath.

Cousins, N. (1976) Anatomy of an Illness. *New England Journal of Medicine* 295: 1458–63.

——(1979) The Holistic Health Explosion. *Saturday Review* 31 March: 17–20.

——(1983) *The Healing Heart*. New York: W.V. Norton.

Cox, H. (1979) *Turning East: The Promise and Peril of the New Orientalism*. New York: Touchstone.

Dossey. L. (1983) *Space, Time, And Medicine*. Boulder: Shambala.

Ehrenreich, J. and Ehrenreich, B. (1970) *The American Health Empire: Power, Profits, and Politics*. New York: Random House.

Ehrenreich, B. and English, D. (1978) *For Her Own Good*. New York: Doubleday & Co.

Ehrenwald, J. (1977) Psi Phenomena and Brain Research. In B. Wolman *Handbook of Parapsychology*. New York: Van Nostrand Rheinhold.

Engel, G. (1977) The Need for a New Medical Model: A Challenge for Biomedicine. *Science* 196: 129–36.

Evans, R.W. (1983) Health Care Technology and the Inevitability of Resource Allocation and Rationing Decisions. *Journal of the American Medical Association*. Part I, 249(15): 2047–53; Part II, 249(16): 2208–222.

Eyer, J. (1984) Capitalism, Health and Illness. In J.B. McKinlay *Issues in the Political Economy of Medical Care*. New York: Methuen. London: Tavistock Publications.

Eyer, J. and Sterling, P. (1977) Stress-related Mortality and Social

Organization. *Review of Radical Political Economics* 9: 1–44.

Ferguson, M. (1978) A New Perspective on Reality. *Mind/Brain Bulletin* 3: 1–4.

Fink, D.L. (1976) Holistic Health: Implications for Health Planning. *American Journal of Health Planning* 1: 23–31.

Flynn, P.A.R. (1980a) *Holistic Health: The Art and Science of Care.* Bowie, MD: Robert Brady.

——(1980b) *The Healing Continuum: Journeys in the Philosophy of Holistic Health.* Bowie, MD: Robert Brady.

Fosshage, J.L. and Olsen, P. (1978) *Healing: Implications for Psychotherapy.* New York: Human Sciences Press.

Frank, J. (1963) *Persuasion and Healing: A Comparative Study of Psychotherapy.* New York: Schocken.

Frankl, V.E. (1955) *Man's Search for Meaning.* New York, Boston: Beacon Press.

——(1965) *The Doctor and the Soul.* New York: Vintage.

Garfield, R. and Salmon, J.W. (1981) Struggles over Health Care in the People's Republic of China. *Journal of Contemporary Asia.* 11: 91–103.

Goddard, J.L. (1973) The Medical Business. *Scientific American* (September): 183–87.

Goldbeck, W.B. (1978) *A Business Perspective on Industry and Health Care.* New York: Springer-Verlag.

Grad, B. (1971–72) Some Biological Effects of "Laying on of Hands." *Journal of Pastoral Counseling* 6: 38–42.

Halifax, J. (1979) *Shamanic Voices: A Survey of Visionary Narratives.* New York: Dutton.

Harman, W. (1981) Science and the Clarification of Values: Implications of Recent Findings in Psychological and Psychic Research. *Journal of Humanistic Psychology* 21: 3–16.

Hastings, A.C., Fadiman, J., and Gordon, J.S. (1980) *Health for the Whole Person.* Boulder, Colorado: Westview Press.

Illich, I. (1976) *Medical Nemesis.* New York: Pantheon.

Joy, W.B. (1979) *Joy's Way.* Los Angeles: J.P. Tarcher.

Kane, R.J. (1980) Iatrogenesis: Just What the Doctor Ordered. *Journal of Community Health* 5: 149–58.

Kaslof, L.J. (1978) *Wholistic Dimensions in Healing.* New York: Doubleday.

Kleinman, A. (1982) Patients Treated by Physicians and Folk Healers: A Comparative Outcome Study in Taiwan. *Culture, Medicine and Psychiatry* 6: 405–23.

Kleinman, A., Kunstadter, P., Alexander, E.R., and Gale, J.L. (1975) *Medicine in Chinese Cultures.* Washington, DC: US Dept. of Health, Education and Welfare Fogarty International Center.

Knowles, J. (1976) *Doing Better, Feeling Worse.* New York: W.W. Norton.

Krieger, D. (1981) *Foundations for Holistic Health Nursing Practices: The Renaissance Nurse*. Philadelphia: J.B. Lippincott.

Krippner, S. and Villoldo, A. (1976) *The Realms of Healing*. Millbrae, CA: Celestial Arts.

Kuhn, T.S. (1962) *The Structure of Scientific Revolutions*. Chicago: University of Chicago Press.

Lambert, E.C. (1978) *Modern Medical Mistakes*. Bloomington: Indiana University Press.

Lampton, D.M. (1974) *Health, Conflict and the Chinese Political System*. Ann Arbor: University of Michigan Press.

——(1977) *The Politics of Medicine in China*. Kent: William Dawon.

LaPatra, J. (1978) *Healing*. New York: McGraw-Hill.

Lasch, C. (1978) *The Culture of Narcissism*. New York: Norton.

Leslie, C. (1976) *Asian Medical Systems*. Berkeley: University of California Press.

Lister, J. (1983) Current Controversy on Alternative Medicine. *The New England Journal of Medicine*. 309: 1524–527.

Manber, M.N. (1978) Chiropractors: Pushing for a Place on the Health Care Team. *Medical World News*, 11 December: 58.

Marti-Ibanez, F. (1960) *Henry E. Sigerist On the History of Medicine*. New York: MD Publications.

McKeown, T. (1971) A Historical Appraisal of the Medical Task. In G. McLachlan and T. KcKeown (eds) *Medical History and Medical Care: A Symposium of Perspectives*. New York: Oxford University Press.

McKinlay, J.B. (1981) From "Promising Report" to "Standard Procedure." *Milbank Memorial Quarterly/Health and Society* 59(3): 374–411.

——(ed.) (1984) *Issues in the Political Economy of Medical Care*. New York: Methuen. London: Tavistock Publications.

McKinlay, J.B. and McKinlay, S. (1977) The Questionable Contribution of Medical Measures to the Decline of Mortality in the United States in the Twentieth Century. *Milbank Memorial Fund Quarterly/Health and Society*. 55: 405–28.

McKinlay, S. and McKinlay, J.B. (1979) Examining Trends in the Nation's Health. Paper presented at the American Public Health Association Annual Meeting, New York, November.

Mechanic, D. (1979) Rationing Medical Care. *The Center Magazine*. September-October: 22–5.

Meek, G. (ed.) (1977) *Healers and the Healing Process*. Wheaton, Ill.: Theosophical Publishing House.

Mendelsohn, R. (1979) *Confessions of a Medical Heretic*. New York: Warner Books.

Menninger, R.W. (1976) Psychiatry 1976: Time for a Holistic Medicine. *Annals of Internal Medicine*. 84: 603–04.

Navarro, V. (1976) *Medicine Under Capitalism*. New York: Prodist.

Needleman, J. and Lewis, D. (1976) *On the Way to Self-Knowledge*. New York: Alfred A. Knopf.

Office of Technology Assessment, US Congress. (1978) *Assessing the Safety and Efficacy of Medical Technologies*. Washington, DC: US Government Printing Office.

Orthodox Medicine, Humanistic Medicine, and Holistic Health (1979–1982) Series of articles in the *Western Journal of Medicine*, beginning 131: 463–65.

Ortiz de Montellano, B. (1975) Empirical Aztec Medicine. *Science* 188: 215–20.

Otto, H.A. and Knight, J.W. (eds) (1979) *Dimensions in Wholistic Healing*. Chicago: Nelson-Hall.

Pelletier, K.R. (1976) *Mind as Healer, Mind as Slayer*. New York: Delta/Delacorte.

——(1979) *Holistic Medicine: From Stress to Optimum Health*. New York: Delcorte Press.

Powles, J. (1973) On the Limitations of Modern Medicine. *Science, Medicine and Man* 1: 1–30.

Reilly, D.T. (1983) Young Doctors' Views on Alternative Medicine. *British Medical Journal* 287: 337–39.

Relman, A.S. (1979) Sounding Board: Holistic Medicine. *The New England Journal of Medicine* 300: 312–13.

——(1980) The New Medical Industrial Complex. *The New England Journal of Medicine* 303: 963–70.

Rogers, M.E. (1980) Nursing: A Science of Unitary Man. In J.P. Riehl and C. Roy *Conceptual Models for Nursing Practice*. New York: Appleton-Century-Crofts.

Rothstein, W. (1972) *American Physicians in the 19th Century*. Baltimore: John Hopkins Press.

Salmon, J.W. (1977) Monopoly Capital and the Reorganization of Health Care. *Review of Radical Political Economics* 9(12): 125–33.

——(1978) *Corporate Attempts to Reorganize the American Health Care System*. Unpublished dissertation, Cornell University.

——(1982) The Competitive Health Strategy: Fighting for Your Health. *Health and Medicine* 1(2): 21–30.

——(1984) Organizing Medical Care for Profit. In J. McKinlay (ed.) *Issues in the Political Economy of Medical Care*. New York: Methuen. London: Tavistock Publications.

Salmon, J.W. and Berliner, H.S. (1980a) The Holistic Health Movement: Challenges to Health Planning. *American Journal of Acupuncture* 8: 197–203.

Salmon, J.W. and Berliner, H.S. (1980b) Health Policy Implications from the Holistic Health Movement. *Journal of Health Politics, Policy and Law* 5(3): 535–53.

Salmon, J.W. and Berliner, H.S. (1982) Self-Care: Boot Straps or Hangman's Noose? *Health and Medicine: Journal of the Health and Medicine Policy Research Group* 1:5–11.

Shryock, R.H. (1936) *The Development of Modern Medicine.* Philadelphia: University of Pennsylvania Press.

——(1960) *Medicine and Society in America, 1660–1860.* New York: New York University Press.

Sidel, V. and Sidel, R. (1972) *Serve the People.* New York: Josiah Macy Foundation.

Sidel, V. and Sidel, R. (1979) *A Healthy State.* New York: Pantheon.

Sigerist, H.E. (1960) The Social History of Medicine. In F. Marti-Ibanez *Henry E. Sigerist On the History of Medicine.* New York: MD Publications.

Smith, T. (1983) Alternative Medicine. *British Medical Journal* 287: 307–08.

Sobel, D.S. (1979) *Ways of Health.* New York: Harcourt Brace Jovanovich.

Stevens, R. (1971) *American Medicine and the Public Interest.* New Haven: Yale University Press.

Totman, R. (1979) *Social Causes of Illness.* New York: Pantheon.

Thomas, L. (1983a) *The Youngest Science: Notes of a Medicine Watcher.* New York: Viking Press.

——(1983b) *Late Night Thoughts to Mahler's Ninth Symphony.* New York: Viking Press.

Turshen, M. (1977) The Political Ecology of Disease. *Review of Radical Political Economics* 9: 45–60.

Waitzkin, H. (1978) A Marxist View of Medical Care. *Annals of Internal Medicine* 89: 264–78.

——(1983) *The Second Sickness: Contradictions of Capitalist Health Care.* New York: Free Press.

Waitzkin, H. and Waterman, B. (1974) *The Exploitation of Illness in Capitalist Society.* Indianapolis: Bobbs-Merrill.

Wartofsky, M. (1975) Organs, Organisms and Disease: Human Ontology and Medical Practice. In H.T. Englehardt, Jr and S. Spicker *Evaluation and Explanation in the Biomedical Sciences.* Boston: D. Reidel.

White, J. (1974) *Psychic Exploration: A Challenge for Science.* New York: Paragon Books.

White, J. and Krippner, S. (1977) *Future Science: Life Energies and the Physics of Paranormal Phenomena.* Garden City, NJ: Anchor/ Doubleday.

Zaretsky, I. and Leone, M. (1972) *Pragmatic Religions: Contemporary Religious Movements in America.* Princeton: Princeton University Press.

Zola, I.K. (1972) Medicine as an Institution of Social Control.

Sociological Review 20: 487–504.

——(1975) In the Name of Health and Illness: On Some Socio-political Consequences of Medical Influence. *Social Science and Medicine* 9: 83–7.

Acknowledgements

My deepest appreciation to Doctors Howard S. Berliner, Daniel Benor, and Agatha M. Gallo for comments on a previous draft. Neither they nor the other authors of this volume should bear any responsibility for the contents of this Introduction.

One

Scientific medicine since Flexner

Howard S. Berliner

Scientific medicine is the generic term for a specific mode of healing characterized by: (1) the assumption that all disease is materially generated by specific etiological agents such as bacteria, viruses, parasites, genetic malformations, or internal chemical imbalances; (2) a passive patient role; and (3) the use of invasive manipulation to restore/maintain the human organism at a statistically derived equilibrium point (health). This mode of healing has been called scientific medicine due to its postulation of rational, as opposed to empirical, theories of disease etiology. It has also been called variously: western medicine, as it originated and predominates in occidental societies; technological medicine, for its extensive reliance on the non-human mediation of illness; and Flexnerian medicine, after Abraham Flexner who popularized this mode of medicine in the United States and Europe at the beginning of the twentieth century.

This chapter will examine the historical development of scientific medicine and attempt to delineate some of the problems with this mode of healing that have led to a search for alternatives.

Scientific medicine emerged in the late nineteenth century

primarily from French and German laboratories (Ackerknecht 1968). It based itself around the discovery of micro-biological agents (bacteria) as the cause of disease and around the theory of specific etiology as a mechanism for explaining the role of these agents. The development of Koch's postulates for the proof of specific causation was a central turning point in this development. It was, however, Edward Lister's discovery of antiseptic technique in surgery in 1867, combined with the discovery of anesthesia twenty years earlier, that gave real impetus to the practical uses of scientific medicine.

Europe, in the mid-nineteenth century, was home to a great number of different theories and practices of medicine. These theories existed a posteriori to the practices which they accompanied, that is, the theories were derivative from the practices – they were empirically derived rather than being inductive in nature (Shryock 1936). Prior to the discovery of bacteria and their implication in the disease process, most theories of disease held the body to be in an imbalance, one that could be remedied by the administration of some chemical or physical force. It is worth noting that as far back as Hippocrates, this had been a common explanation for disease. The medical practice of the nineteenth century modes of healing was dependent on the intake of foodstuffs, drugs, chemicals, vapors, the administration of hot or cold water, or exposure to the elements. It should also be noted that the morbidity of the time was such that most disease was self-limiting and life span short. Medicine was largely irrelevant to the process of healing (as it is understood today in scientific medicine) except in those cases where it was harmful enough to cause morbidity or mortality itself, which was apparently quite frequently (Duffy 1979).

Beginning in Europe in the 1850s and in the US a decade later, was the sanitary revolution that led to environmental reforms affecting drinking water, sewerage, housing and work conditions. The sanitary revolution was the offshoot of theories of medicine that looked toward social, political, and environmental factors as a breeding ground for disease (rather than as a disease in itself) (Rosen 1958). There is a great deal of evidence to suggest that it was the sanitary revolution more than anything else, that did much to lower mortality rates and lengthen life expectancy in the late nineteenth century (Powles 1973;

McKinlay and McKinlay 1977). It was thus in the context of an unheralded but noticeable decline in mortality and morbidity that the foundation of what was to be called scientific medicine arose.

Scientific medicine was distinguished from competing modes of healing in several ways: (1) its understanding of the basis of disease, as explained above; (2) its class specific practitioner base; (3) its research orientation; and (4) its location of practice (Berliner 1977). Scientific medicine demanded a special formal education of its practitioners. This stood it in marked contrast to other medical practices which required only the barest minimums of education and an apprenticeship with a medical practitioner for a medical degree. Thus scientific medicine was able to limit future practitioners to those who could afford to undertake the long and arduous training demanded (financially more than physically). In essence this limited scientific medical physicians to upper and upper-middle class citizens. Scientific medicine was also different in that its basis was research rather than empirical practice. In part because it was limited to the wealthy who were independent of the financial need to make a living in medical practice and in part because its leaders were, for the most part, salaried academics, it could devote itself to the luxury of research and the development of theory. It should be noted that when clinical examination did take place, its site was generally the hospital rather than the patient's home or the physician's office where other healers plied their trade. As the next section shall indicate these differences were not insignificant.

The initial clinical advances made under the banner of scientific medicine came in the field of surgery. Based on Joseph Lister's application of bacteriological insights to the operating table (antisepsis), along with the prior discovery of general anesthesia and numerous technical advances in equipment, surgery became the major growth center of medicine in the 1880s. Safe, effective surgery did much to increase the popular enthusiasm for medicine. At the same time, the discovery of the etiology of numerous diseases in discrete bacteria also helped to focus popular attention on this emerging mode of medicine. It is especially important to note that on a statistical level virtually none of these advances in bacteriology and related sciences had any impact upon the treatment of disease in humans until the 1930s. A few specific exceptions were smallpox and diphtheria. While individual treatments may have been significant, overall mortality and morbidity rates were already in decline. The reasons for this decline have been assumed to be improved nutritional status and the public health improvements noted above. As McKeown and others have noted the contribution of scientific medicine, to the decline in mortality rates, was not significant until the second quarter of this century, by which time the larger proportion of the total decline in mortality had already been achieved (McKeown 1971). As Powles further notes:

> it is widely believed that the introduction of antibiotics and effective immunization campaigns marked a dramatic breakthrough in the fight against infectious diseases. Whilst this may have been true in particular cases – for example, immunization against diphtheria, – their contribution to the total decline in mortality over the last two centuries has been a minor one. Most of the reduction had already occurred before they were introduced and there was only a slight downward inflection in an otherwise declining curve following their introduction.   (Powles 1973: 7)

Nevertheless, scientific medicine was given credit for dramatic breakthroughs and received much popular and institutional support for further work. Scientific medicine grew in different ways. In Europe the creation of state supported research institutes became the dominant mechanism for obtaining new medical findings. Such renowned centers as the Lister Institute, the Pasteur Institute, and the Koch Institute were named after major figures of scientific medicine and in many cases were generously supported by an admiring public.

   In the US little was done in the way of medical research until the 1890s. Most Americans interested in studying scientific medicine went to Europe to study in one of the research laboratories. It has been estimated that over 15,000 Americans travelled to Europe to study medicine between 1890 and 1915 (Bonner 1963). In 1893 the Johns Hopkins School of Medicine was opened, the first center for scientific medicine research and education in the United States. In 1901, the Rockefeller Institute for Medical Research was opened in New York, the first privately endowed research center in the US. It is noteworthy that the Rockefeller had to import most of its research scientists from Europe as there were not enough Americans trained to undertake advanced research in the US at this time (Corner 1965). Over the next few years, literally dozens of privately endowed research institutes were opened in the US following the Rockefeller lead and spurred on by its example.

American medicine at the turn of the century was dominated by practitioners of allopathic medicine. The allopaths outnumbered the next largest leading practitioner group, homoeopaths, by ten to one (Rothstein 1968). Dozens of other modalities of medicine were practiced in the US by large numbers of independent healers. The educational standards for all types of medicine were not particularly high. Much medical education was obtained in proprietary medical schools of far from rigorous standards. American physicians represented the population at large in that all classes and races had access to some form of medical education and credentialing or certification. The transition to a research-oriented scientific medicine had its main impact in the US in the alteration of the social and class composition of the physician population (Berliner 1975). The vehicle for this transformation was the Flexner Report of 1910, a report on medical education in the US and Canada (Flexner 1910). The Flexner Report exposed the scandalous conditions in North American medical schools and advocated a scientific medicine patterned on the Johns Hopkins plan, which itself was modeled on the German medical education system. This meant, in essence, that prior to medical education, potential students would be required to have both a high school and a four-year college diploma. Medical school itself would be four years followed by a year-long hospital based clinical internship. During the medical schooling, the first two years would be spent largely in laboratories studying the basic sciences and anatomy while the last two years would be spent on the hospital wards. Over the next twenty-five years, over $600 million was spent changing American medical education to fit this model (Berliner 1977). While the large American philanthropic foundations were the prime vehicles for the financing of this change (almost $100 million from the Rockefeller philanthropies alone), private contributions and public fund-raising also supported this educational reform. It is thus fair to say that after 1910, scientific medicine became institutionalized as the dominant mode of medicine in the US. Similarly, in the UK and Europe, American foundations, led by the Rockefeller philanthropies, gave considerable financial assistance to the rebuilding of medical schools that had been damaged during World War I. The principle was the same as in the American educational reforms, with support going primarily to research institutions devoted to the pursuit of scientific medicine.

The immediate results of the Flexner reforms were highly visible in the US. Of the 131 medical schools that were in operation in 1900, only 95 were operating in 1915 and only 81 remained by 1922. This continued a trend which had started well before Flexner and owed much to the declining economic positions of the schools in a depressed American economy (particularly the recession of 1907–09). The number of new physicians produced annually fell from 5,700 per year in 1900 to 2,300 per year in 1919 (Sheps and Lewis 1983). Of greater importance than the aggregate decline in the number of schools and graduates was the change in the student body composition of the remaining schools. The necessity for a college degree and the four-year curriculum allowed only upper-class students to continue to study medicine. The ability of people with limited financial means to become physicians was severely restricted. For example, of the seven medical schools that specifically trained blacks to be physicians, five were closed. All five medical schools which specifically trained women to be physicians were closed. The schools that remained began a shift towards a scientific orientation in which the hospital became the center of educational focus and research became the dominant activity.

Scientific medicine was not just a new name for Allopathy, although many allopaths adopted the framework and terminology of the new medicine in an attempt to appropriate the legitimacy conferred by the name scientific medicine. It is important to stress this point as it has created a considerable confusion among historians. Scientific medicine had a different theoretical basis and epistemology than other existing modes of medicine of the late nineteenth and early twentieth century, but it had an extremely limited clinical and therapeutic repertoire (Berliner 1983). In its early period scientific medicine was a unique way of organizing the clinical experience, but it was not, at that time, a clinical medicine. The leading scientific medicine clinician of the time, William Osler (of Johns Hopkins and later Oxford), advocated allopathic therapies for conditions that had been diagnosed through scientific means because there were no scientific remedies for these problems. Since the research program of scientific medicine had not yet produced a significant number of clinically effective outcomes, public support for scientific medicine was based on the success of science in endeavors other than medicine. It was a faith in science and what that word implied, much more than an implicit belief in this new mode of medicine that led to its public acceptance. As Daniels notes:

> Nothing was more important to that [age] than "science." It was a word to conjure with, a word to sweep away all opposition by labelling it "benighted," "romantic," or "obscurantist;" a word to legitimize any program no matter what fundamental reorganizations it might entail or what sacrifices it might call upon particular groups to make. . . . If the "science" involved . . . seldom possesses the rigor of a Newtonian Law, few would notice, the name had a magic of its own that made questioning irrelevant. . . . Technology especially fired Americans' imaginations giving them unlimited hopes for the future. [They] were increasingly impressed by the visible manifestations of the power of technology that had appeared at an accelerating rate since the third quarter of the nineteenth century . . . the telephones, telegraphs and electric lights . . . were more powerful arguments from that layman's point of view than was the most elegant theorem of mathematical physics.
>
> (Daniels 1971:289–91)

If scientific medicine could not deliver, it could certainly promise. The news of every new discovery was trumpeted around the globe, even when those discoveries might have little or no applicability to the treatment of actual problems. The discovery of rabies vaccine was widely heralded as a victory for scientific medicine and mankind, but rabies was a rare disease and the vaccine was often ineffective. Andrew Carnegie set up a fund to send American children with rabies to the Pasteur Institute to obtain treatment there. The newspapers and magazines followed the send-offs very closely, but rarely followed up on the outcome of the trip. Similarly, diphtheria antitoxin was largely ineffective when it was first introduced into the US, but the newspaper and magazine reader of the day would not have known that from the media attention that it received. The discovery of the bacterial causes of a disease did not immediately presage the discovery of a cure for that disease, although that hope was always present. A case in point came in 1902 with the discovery of the parasitical cause of hookworm disease. A New York newspaper loudly proclaimed with a banner headline: "GERM OF LAZINESS FOUND," giving the impression that even those conditions thought to be social conditions rather than disease states could be remedied through scientific medicine (Berliner 1977). This was not an isolated example of the media marketing through hyperbole. As late as 1923, Frederick T. Gates, responsible for all the Rockefeller philanthropic giving, could say:

> Disease is the supreme ill of human life and it is the main source of almost all other human ills, poverty, ignorance, vice, inefficiency, hereditary taint and many other evils.
>
> (Gates 1923)

The implication being that more research was needed to find the biological origins of these "diseases" and that cures would result shortly thereafter. The financial support given to scientific medicine was not matched by support for competing modes of healing. Except for those modalities which had broad-based popular and financial strength (such as chiropractic, osteopathy, and Christian Science) other modes of medicine were swept aside in the great public onrush of support for scientific medicine.

An analogy may help explain the public reaction to scientific medicine. In the 1980s we are told that the personal computer is the wave of the future and that our lives will become totally dependent upon computers in the next few years. While there is little that the computer can do right now that is of interest or use to the ordinary individual, people have been rushing out to buy them so as not to be unprepared for the future. I would argue that scientific medicine held a similar promise and a similar lack of personal utility around the turn of the century, but that people still wanted to be part of its movement. The same factors clearly held true for physicians and other healers who may have seen in scientific medicine, if not in the support for scientific medicine, the wave of the future.

The period from 1920 to the 1950s has been called the "watershed of American medicine" by Ivan Illich (Illich 1976). By this is meant that in this period American medicine had its most successful and popular span. It was during this period that the most dramatic declines in mortality and morbidity rates were recorded and in this period that longevity and life expectancy took on modern dimensions. There were vast improvements in clinical medicine and the continued development of surgical skills. The development of mass produced pharmaceuticals and especially antibiotics and the improved technology for blood transfusion, along with such devices as the electrocardiograph and the electroencephalograph. There were improved vaccines for such diseases as polio and the mass development of relatively safe radiographic equipment. All these factors helped to increase the confidence of the populace in American medicine, now synonymous with scientific medicine. The numbers of American scientists winning prestigious international awards for medical discoveries and advances became a symbol of how far American research capacity had increased since the turn of the century. In the period following World War II large numbers of foreign students began to come to America to study medicine, as large numbers of Americans had gone to the centers of new discovery in Europe only a few decades before. In popular terms, this was the period in which the first significant fruits of scientific medicine actually reached the population at large. Nevertheless, the clinical and technological breakthroughs were not always translatable into bedside medicine for all Americans. Germany had instituted a national sickness insurance in the 1880s and Britain instituted national health insurance in 1911. After World War II most European countries had universal health insurance schemes allowing all residents access to medical care services. Britain had gone as far as instituting a National Health Service in 1948. The United States did not follow suit in this regard, relying on a voluntary health insurance system that individuals purchased through employment.

Beginning in the post World War II period, access to scientific medicine became a problem for large numbers of Americans. The elderly, especially the unemployed elderly, and the poor groups that utilize a disproportionate share of medical care resources were without the financial means to obtain needed care. This was a problem that was now new, but had taken on increased dimension as medical technology and developments drove up the costs of medical care. The problem was given prominence as a significant national problem with the rediscovery of poverty in America in the early 1960s (Berliner 1973).

The period of the 1960s was one in which there was a tremendous expansion of access to scientific medicine. The passage of acts entitling elderly and poor Americans to medical care paid for by the government was a tremendous advance for the large numbers of these people who had been denied medical care. The costs of providing this care were far higher than had been imagined, and this along with the venality of health care providers, forced the costs of care up so high, that by the end of the decade, the President of the US could declare a crisis in health care financing in the country (Salmon 1975). It should be noted that the 1960s was the period of "guns and butter" in the US when the country was trying to increase both military spending and social spending at the same time with no increases in revenue. By the start of the 1970s, a retrenchment from the open-ended entitlement programs had begun, still continuing in the 1980s with cutbacks of access and benefits (Berliner and Salmon 1979). The Reagan administration has promoted the use of competition between competing providers of health care to attempt to lower health care costs, an effort which has exacerbated the tendency of proprietization of health care services in the US (Salmon 1982). There is much current discussion of the medical-industrial complex, and proprietary chains now own over one-sixth of all US hospital beds (Relman 1980). These financial problems reflect changes in the nature of medical care which emanate from the dominant principles and postulates of scientific medicine. This is to say that medicine, and any other social process, is greatly influenced by the political-economic context in which it exists. The mode of medicine that is dominant in a period of late capitalism begins to take on some aspects of that system (Berliner 1983).

The mainstreams of popular discontent with, and awareness of, the limitations of the medical model stem from a variety of factors which, when linked together, provide a trenchant critique of modern medical care. These factors include: (1)

changes in the disease structure of modern societies; (2) changes in demographic patterns; (3) changes in the patient-physician relationship; (4) the limitations of the hospital; (5) problems associated with the technological approach to medicine; (6) the problems associated with the machine model orientation of scientific medicine; (7) the focus on cure over prevention in research and practice; and (8) the cost of medical care.

Changing disease structure

The initial focus of scientific medicine in the 1890s was on diseases of bacterial and parasitic origin, as these were the only specific agents of causation known at the time. As I have argued above, it is not at all clear that scientific medicine *per se* deserves the credit for eliminating the disease conditions that surrounded it during its early years, but nevertheless very few of the diseases present at the turn of the century are serious medical problems today in the US. Of the leading causes of death in 1900, only heart disease and cancer remain as the leading causes in 1980 (World Almanac 1904, 1983). Most of the credit for this dramatic change in the disease structure must go to the public health and sanitary reform movement. What we can see in the changing patterns of mortality over the past 80 to 100 years has been: (1) a significant shift toward diseases affecting people at older ages, and concomitantly a significant drop in the infant mortality rate; (2) a marked increase in mortality that may not be biological in origin, e.g. accidents and suicide; and (3) an extremely large increase in deaths from diseases which may have a strong social component and a multifactorial etiology, e.g. cancer, heart disease, cirrhosis, and arteriosclerosis. The exclusive focus of scientific medicine research on the biological, to the virtual exclusion of the non- somatic, the social, and the environmental, has been well documented (Berliner and Salmon 1980). Another evident fact in the mortality data is the overall decline in death rates over'the last eighty years. In 1900 the age adjusted total death rate from all causes was 17.8 deaths per 1,000 population. In 1980 it has been reduced to 5.9 deaths per 1,000 population (DH + HS 1980: 159). Moreover, the differences in death rates by age show an increasing male mortality rate peaking in 1970 and more recently a gradual decline in the difference between men and women. This may be due to a notable decline in male mortality from heart disease and simultaneous increase in female deaths from cancer. Another clear fact that emerges from any study of mortality data in the US is based around the social epidemiology of illness. Non-whites in the US who have less access to the fruits of civilization, including medical care, have markedly higher death rates at all ages than do whites. What we may be witnessing in the US in the 1980s is a shift in public demand for modes of healing better able to give the above noted factors more prominence in their theoretical models and practice.

In general the alternatives to scientific medicine tend to focus to a greater degree on chronic disease palliation and thus place themselves more in touch with consumer demands than scientific medicine.

Changing demographic patterns

Although people who are over sixty-five have only a slightly longer life expectancy now than they did in 1900 (11.9 years then against 16.3 years now), people born today have a 25.9 year longer life expectancy than people born in 1900 (DH + HS 1980: 131). This is to say that the vast majority of the reduction in mortality has taken place in the lowest age brackets. While people who reach old age do not live substantially longer than they did at the turn of the century, there are a significantly greater number of people reaching old age. Thus there is a projected 30 per cent increase in the number of people who will be over sixty-five in the US between 1975 and the year 2000, a 71 per cent increase in the number of people over eighty-five. By the year 2030, it is projected that 18.3 per cent of the US population will be over sixty-five, a doubling of this population in the past fifty years (Grana 1982). This is significant because "the elderly are more likely than any other age group to be hospitalized, stay longer in the hospital and to consume more physician visits and prescription drugs per capita" (Grana 1982: 105–6). The per capita spending on health care is nearly three times higher for the elderly than for the population as a whole.

Moreover the elderly suffer primarily from chronic conditions, defined by the Office of the Assistant Secretary for Planning and Evaluation of the Department of Health and Human Services in 1981 as "those in which nonreversible pathological alterations or congenital defects cause residual disability which requires habilitation, rehabilitation, supervision and care over a long period of time" (DH + HS 1981). The essence of these statistics reveals that the demography of the US is changing in such a way as to produce a great increase in the numbers of elderly people who suffer from health care problems that are not presently amenable to treatment by scientific medicine. It should be noted that the aging of the population is more than just an American phenomenon, with similar changes occurring in European nations as well. In Great Britain, for example, the percentage of the population over sixty-five has increased from 4.7 per cent in 1901 to 11.7 per cent in 1961, to 15.0 per cent in 1981, and is projected to be 14.0 per cent of the population in the year 2001. The reason for the decline between 1981 and 2001 is due to the reduced population cohort due to World War II. Nevertheless, between 1981 and 2001, the population of Great Britain over eighty-five will increase by 50 per cent and the population over seventy-five will increase by 8 per cent (Jefferies 1983). Alternatives to scientific medicine tend to focus their efforts on the alleviation of pain and the involvement of patients in their own care and have spurned the use of hospital-based high technology services, so that they are usually less expensive than scientific medical treatment.

Relation of the patient to the physician

Specialists, physicians, and other healers who limit their ministrations to one particular part of the body or disease syndrome have existed as far back as ancient Egypt. Nevertheless, most physicians until the era of scientific medicine have been generalists in the sense that they treated all patients that they saw. Scientific medicine encouraged physicians to do research and the expertise gained in this endeavor, and the vast amount of knowledge accumulated, led them to specialize their practice to the organ system, part of the body or disease that they studied. The result of this increase in specialization has been to deprive the patient of a physician who can look at him or her as a whole person. Scientific medicine creates a hierarchy in which research scientists and practitioners in specialty medical fields have greater prestige, status, and material rewards than do those in general medical practice. This has led, in the US to the overproduction of specialty physicians and the under-production of general care doctors. Note that the US system differs from that of the UK in that all physicians have access to a hospital and there is no technical or social distinction between doctors who practice in the hospital and those who don't. Because the US lacks a comprehensive health care system, such as exists in the UK, most Americans receive their treatment at either the physician's office, or increasingly the hospital, at their discretion. The care that most people need most of the time is called primary care. Primary care, of necessity, must view the body in a holistic manner, that is, it must take all bodily and emotional symptoms into account when examining the patient. Because scientific medicine concentrates on parts of the body, rather than the whole body, it is implicitly biased against primary care medicine. Moreover, the nature of training in an academic medical center makes the provision of routine care seem boring.

Because of the specialty approach to medicine, a person will generally require the services of several different physicians during a lifetime. Therefore, the ability to have a physician who is intimately familiar with a person's background and history is severely hampered. A typical female, for example, will start with a pediatrician, graduate to an internist and an obstetrician/ gynecologist, pick up a pediatrician for her children and still have need for a dermatologist or an oncologist. For all of these physicians, the patients will present as a stranger and any information that the physician has will come from a standard history form. The mobility of Americans being what it is, few people retain any serial relationship with a particular physician for very long, and it is extremely rare to hear of a person who uses the physician that their parents used.

Scientific medicine encourages passivity on the part of the patient. This tendency has been explained under the rubric of ''sick role theory'' in medical sociology (Susser and Watson 1971). The essence of this theory is that as part of the social contract, a person claiming to be ill is exempted from their normal social role (going to school, going to work, etc.), if the physician concurs with the claim and if they allow the physician to minister to them. Scientific medicine is perhaps the only mode of healing that demands virtual passivity on the part of the patient. This is based on the postulate of scientific medicine that accepts only somatic data as being valid for judgment-making on the part of the physician. Thus patients in systems of scientific medicine are more or less forced to surrender themselves to largely unknown physicians who will treat them completely independent of their social history (Wartofsky 1975).

The training that physicians receive under scientific medicine is almost exclusively devoted to dealing with disease, as opposed to keeping people healthy. The reasons for this are that: (1) scientific medicine assumes that a person is healthy until he or she becomes sick – its understanding of health is the absence of identifiable disease; and (2) because scientific medical training is based around the hospital, where the patients are presumably sick, the physician rarely gets to see healthy people or find out in what circumstances they best retain their health. Much criticism has been given to scientific medicine for ignoring epidemiology in the training of medical students, and this criticism could be applied to ignoring psychology, nutrition, environmental and occupational health, as well. It fails to see these fields as important relative to pharmacology or genetics.

Alternatives to scientific medicine have focused on fostering a relationship between the patient and the healer and involving the patient in the healing process. The notion of a passive patient is explicitly rejected and the patient is encouraged to participate in defining symptoms and evaluating therapy. It is important to note that many alternative medicines utilize a specialty type approach towards illness, by utilizing only one therapeutic technique or one diagnostic methodology. These alternatives cannot be considered holistic.

The limitations of the hospital

Advocates of scientific medicine claim that the location of disease treatment in the hospital was a major advance in the conquest of human illness. Indeed, the hospital allows for the centralization and standardization of disease diagnosis and treatment. It was the use of the hospital that propelled scientific medicine rather than vice versa. While there have been obvious benefits in having the hospital serve as the locus of medical care, there have been major problems associated with this as well. The major effect that hospital-based medical care has on the diagnostic process is to render the patient anonymous by stripping him or her of social identity (Berliner 1977). When people enter the hospital they are removed from familiar ethnic/occupational/environmental/cultural/social/familial/geographic surroundings, dressed alike in hospital gowns and fed the same food. Whatever role these factors might play in the disease process is intentionally removed. Since many of these factors have been implicated in the chronic diseases that form the bulk of the disease burden in western society, the utility of this process seems questionable (Eyer 1975). Yet, scientific medicine does not recognize these social factors as part of its understanding of the disease process. By not allowing for the social mediation of disease, hospitals are not as effective as they could potentially be and they increase the costs of medical care. The invasive procedures utilized by scientific medicine require long periods of convalescence and recuperation, often completely disconnected from the patients' support network and historic routine. There is a clear need to keep the beds filled and the equipment in use, independent of the actual needs of the patients. It has been noted that there is far more surgery and diagnostic testing in the US than the health status of this country would seem to mandate (US OTA 1978). The US has twice the rate of surgery of the UK and there is no apparent difference in the health of people in the two countries.

Alternatives to scientific medicine have for the most part not favored hospital-based care. Most use a practitioner's office to render their services. Most alternatives also directly try to include the social universe of their patients in their treatment. This is particularly true in those medicines that are culturally or folk-ways based.

Technology

The counter-culture of the 1960s led many Americans to explicitly reject techology and the technological orientation of modern life. Many no longer believe, as they once did, that the answer to all the problems of today can be found, and certainly not through new developments, scientific discoveries, or technological breakthroughs. The illusion of control that Americans thought they had over their destiny was ultimately shattered with the OPEC oil crisis of 1973. The need to depend on other nations for their products was brought home to the American people in a most immediate way. Americans were either forced out of economic necessity, or saw benefits, to conserve energy. Other facets of their dependence soon became clear. The publication of *Medical Nemesis* by Ivan Illich in 1974, helped to raise discussion of people's dependence upon physicians and their medicine. A conscious attempt by people to decrease their dependence on medical care ensued and was manifested in discussions of the limited efficacy and safety of scientific medicine and the role of personal risk factors in preventing illness. Taking the form of self-care and individualistic nutrition and exercise programs, the need for an external medical care system became problematic for many. Women, in particular, began to challenge the control over their bodies exercised by medicine and physicians, and to reject non-holistic formulations (Frankfort 1973). The birth control pill was criticized for example because male-dominated medicine had discounted the deleterious health effects it had on women. Other gynecological and reproductive practices were similarly scrutinized and criticized. The failure of scientific medicine to find cures for the leading causes of death and disability has also given new impetus to the search for alternative practices. The problems associated with the major weapons that scientific medicine uses against disease – radiation, chemotherapy, and surgery – have led many to seek less harmful alternatives, much as the risks of allopathy drove people into the safer arms of homoeopathy and alternative practitioners in the later nineteenth century (Rothstein 1968).

Scientific medicine has built its armamentarium of technology to diagnose and treat illness and disease. As noted above, scientific medicine is based on the use of invasive techniques to combat disease. In this combat, the risk of iatrogenesis – medical system induced disease or disability – is immense. Many diagnostic procedures used in scientific medicine are risky in that they threaten to either kill or disable the patient. In many cases morbidity and mortality result from the inappropriate use of technologies. A case in point would be the use of mass screening for breast cancer through X-raying large numbers of women at a time. It has been observed that the use of X-rays may actually induce breast cancer rather than just detect it. A similar case might be the pernicious effects of cancer chemotherapy on other parts of the body, independent of its effect on the cancer it is supposed to be aimed at. There are other forms of iatrogenesis as well. When a surgeon removes the wrong organ or nicks an organ with a surgical instrument, that is also iatrogenesis. When a physician prescribes a drug in the wrong dose or prescribes the wrong drug, that too is iatrogenesis.

Iatrogenesis is only one side of the technology issue, the other is ineffectiveness. Very few of the techniques of scientific medicine have been clinically evaluated. Many common, everyday procedures still used by scientific medicine are carryovers from allopathic medicine that have never been rigorously tested. It is not surprising then to find that when the techniques of scientific medicine are evaluated, many turn out to be no more effective than a placebo, and some to be actually harmful (US OTA 1978). The high cost of modern technology, its potential iatrogenic effects combined with its potential lack of efficacy have created much public outcry. While people are desirous of technologies that will make them healthy or healthier, at almost any price, people are loath to invest scarce dollars in useless, harmful equipment.

In the late 1970s, American hospitals became interested in the CAT scanner, a British import that cost over $500,000 to buy and a similar amount to operate. Before there was any formal assessment of the utility of this new technology, almost every university hospital attempted to buy one. As it turned out, clinical uses for the CAT scanner did emerge in time, and it is now a welcome addition to most hospitals' diagnostic capacity, but it seems more luck than anything else that it turned out that way. American hospitals are constantly in the throes of technological acquisition. A recent advance is the Nuclear Magnetic Resonance scanner, a cousin to the CAT scanner. The NMR scanner is theoretically safer than the CAT scanner as it does not use radiation, but it requires a special installation in a specially constructed room. The costs for this new technology are in the millions, rather than the hundreds of thousands.

A similar story could be told about the growth in use of the fetal monitor, growth which has occurred in the UK as well as the US (Day 1982). The fetal monitor was developed to follow the heartbeat of the fetus as its mother went through labor. If any fetal distress was detected, if the fetal heart stopped beating, for example, the obstetrician could perform an immediate caesarian section on the woman and save the fetus. It was intended that this monitoring would be restricted to high-risk pregnancies, those in which it was feared that something would go wrong. Nevertheless, once in the hospital the equipment tended to be used, and if no high-risk deliveries presented themselves, it was used on normal deliveries. Many woman had negative reactions to the new equipment. Not only did it scare them, but they misunderstood its function. They assumed that if this was being used on them, their infants must be in trouble and this created a great deal of psychic distress. Of even more concern was the fact that whenever there was an indication of any sort of fetal distress, the obstetricians began to stop the normal delivery and begin the caesarian delivery. In some cases, the fetal distress was a temporary anomaly of the birth process; in some cases it was a direct result of the distress the mother was in. In any event, the net effect of the use of fetal monitors has been to markedly increase the number of caesarian deliveries in hospitals. Since the risk of iatrogenesis is increased so greatly in this type of birth, and the costs are so much higher, this potentially helpful piece of technology has become a prime factor in increased morbidity and cost.

The alternatives to scientific medicine tend to be non-technological in orientation and non-invasive in approach. They tend to utilize and to stress the human mediation of illness, rather than the technological. In most cases, the Alternative medicines, when they do use technological approaches, tend to use them with somewhat more discretion and with less emphasis on the therapeutic process than scientific medicine.

The machine model

The basis for scientific medical research is the assumption that the body consists of a large number of independent, though functionally related, systems each of which can be studied discretely. Further underlying this assumption is the belief that the somatic functions of the body are independent of the mind. This belief is a mainstay of the cartesian materialism upon which science based itself in the seventeenth century and has become the most obvious and most anomalous critique of scientific medicine in recent times. In its most simple formulation, scientific medicine maintains that each cell in the body functions solely on the basis of its genetic instructions and that external influences have little effect on the behavior of the cell, except in so far as they can alter or mutate genetic information or penetrate the cell wall and do damage to the cell. Given this operating principle, it is difficult for scientific medicine to explain any relationship between mental states and physical functions. Yet much of the modern disease burden seems to have a psychological component, in that the psychological state of a person can exert a great influence over the acquisition or even severity of an illness. Other non-physically based factors are similarly excluded from significant consideration as potential agents of disease causation or generation. These include social, environmental, occupational, and stress-related factors.

Another result of the machine model approach is the belief that almost anything can be done to any one organ or part of the body – it can be replaced, modified, removed – without having an effect on other parts of the body. Thus the modern mania for transplants of all sorts and the penchant for heroic operations that preserve a segment of body functioning at the expense of consciousness or quality of life. Again this has been the cause of a severe public backlash, because while the possibility of longer life is intriguing and a clear public good, the quality of the life that results from these mediations of the physical processes of the body is at odds with modern conceptions of what the quality of life should be. For example, children who are born with a genetic deficiency that turns off their immune system would normally die within a few weeks or months. Scientists have found that by keeping the children in plastic tents or domes with bacteria and viruses filtered out of the air, the children could seemingly live forever – their immune systems no longer mattered as they were externally protected from harmful agents. So, a mechanism exists to allow science to bypass a defect of the body. But the real effect of this action is to force these children to live their entire lives within this tent, never touching another human being, never leaving this artificial cocoon. More recently, an elderly dentist who would have died in a few weeks from chronic heart disease, was given an artificial heart. He was kept tethered to a large machine that kept the artificial heart functioning, but rarely got out of bed during the several months of this experiment, until he died. While his body may have been kept alive a few additional weeks by this mechanism, did he really live those weeks, as humans ordinarily understand that term? These issues and others like them have spawned a new field, known as bio-ethics, which deals with such problems as who should get transplants, given that more people need them than are organs available; when should heroic measures be ended, if ever; when should people be allowed to die; what does the term death mean?

Alternatives to scientific medicine focus on the unity of the mind and the body and the essential connections between organ systems and the external environment, broadly constructed. Death is not generally construed as a failure of medicine to be avoided at all costs in most alternatives, but rather as a natural end to the life cycle that can be understood by people when placed in a relevant social context. Thus death with dignity and death surrounded by family and friends is portrayed as an alternative approach to scientific medicine's technological life.

Cure and prevention

As noted earlier in this chapter, scientific medicine strives primarily to cure and only marginally to prevent. Since it assumes a state of health until some detectable (physical) illness or symptom appears, it has no way of relating to prevention. To the extent that it bases itself upon a mode of epidemiology which assumes a single specific cause (the doctrine of specific etiology), the notion of multiple causality or indirect causation is not considered. A magic bullet mentality thus ensues in which all research is aimed at finding the single specific cause and cure of a disease. This may have had some utility when diseases clearly had a single cause and were amenable to a single cure, and it was certainly fostered by the development of antibiotics, but it does not seem to work very well for chronic diseases and where the main need is for palliation and rehabilitation, areas that are virtually ignored by scientific medicine. It should be noted that scientific medicine is not solely to blame for this state of affairs, the system of medical care delivery also being a great influence. There is far more emphasis on prevention in the UK than in the US due to the National Health Service of the former and the fee for service orientation of the latter.

Alternatives to scientific medicine focus on prevention of illness and the maintenance of health. Prevention is understood to be the process of keeping the person in the best possible state of well-being that the person is capable of sustaining. Preventive orientation tends to revolve around diet, exercise, mental state, and affirmative sense of self. It is not that scientific medical therapy does not encourage these orientations, but rather that they do not represent the main thrust of where the major emphasis of scientific medicine is placed.

Cost

More than any other issue, it has been the high cost of scientific medical care that has led to questions of its efficacy and safety in its approach to health. Because of its use of highly trained practitioners and its emphasis on high technology diagnostic and curative procedures, it has become a very expensive mode of healing. A stay in the hospital for the most routine of problems runs into the thousands of dollars, and should there be a need for anything exotic, bills in the hundreds of thousands of dollars result. For this reason the amount of the Gross National Product spent on health services in the US is over 10 per cent. The costs of health care have been increasing by roughly 15 per cent per year, even when inflation in other sectors of the economy has abated. The high cost of medical care has cut off millions of Americans, who do not have a national health insurance or national health service, from medical care. Many Americans who have either lost access to medical care services, or never had it, or who have been unable to afford care, have turned to alternative modes of healing and self-care.

Alternatives to scientific medicine tend to be relatively less expensive, as they do not utilize high technology services or hospitalization and tend to rely on natural, easy-to-obtain substances when they use drugs at all. While cost should not be a major factor in deciding the mode of healing used in a society, it has become one of the major factors in western countries. The US has been attempting, unsuccessfully, to cut down the cost of medical care since 1969. The Reagan administration is more aggressive in its actual and planned reductions of benefits and payments than prior administrations have been. In the UK, the National Health Service has been losing total budget and staff due to the declining British economy.

Conclusions

As the other chapters in this book make evident, scientific medicine is under assault from a wide spectrum of alternative healing practices. Some of these pose legitimate threats to the hegemony of scientific medicine, others do not. All are testimony to the increasing public disaffection with modern medicine and its associated delivery system. The centrality of the medical enterprise to modern economies is such that it is unlikely that major changes will occur quickly. Far more likely is the probability that scientific medicine will absorb and co-opt changes from the outside, and perhaps gradually evolve into a different medicine. A good example of this process is the case of acupuncture. In the wake of the normalization of relations between the US and mainland China in the early 1970s, much public interest was generated by the Chinese practice of acupuncture. The media reported in glowing terms on the success of surgical operations performed only under acupuncture anesthesia, and many American medical teams went to China to study this phenomenon and brought back first-hand reports as well. It quickly became a major fad in affluent urban settings to have an acupuncturist to deal with a variety of medical and quasi-medical problems. There were only two problems with this: scientific medicine had no way of reconciling acupuncture meridiens with current neurological explanations of pain abatement; and acupuncture was being performed by people who were not medical doctors – a veritable stream of money was being lost to the profession (Kaptchuk 1983). In most states in the US the situation was remedied by allowing acupuncture to be performed only under the supervision of licensed medical doctors. Rather than becoming an alternative modality in and of itself, it was brought under the wing of scientific medicine even though its epistemology was completely at odds with that espoused by scientific medicine. It was co-opted. This co-optation process is likely to continue along with the simultaneous rejection of all alternatives as quackery and charlatanism. The challenge from potential rivals can be taken seriously and dealt with in a hostile manner, as in a recent "Sounding Board" article in the *New England Journal of Medicine*:

> If holistic health advocates were content with encouraging sensible preventive medicine or with criticizing the economic organization of American medicine, we might be enthusiastic, but they are not. If the movement were without influence on American life, we would be indifferent, but it is not. Holistic medicine is a pabulum of common sense and nonsense offered by cranks and quacks and failed pedants who share an attachment to magic and an animosity toward reason. Too many people seem willing to swallow the rhetoric – even too many medical doctors – and the results will not be benign. At times, physicians may find themselves in sympathy with the holistic movement, because some fragment of the rhetoric rings true, because of certain practices and attitudes they encounter in their daily work with colleagues and patients, or because of dissatisfaction with the economic and social organization of medicine. One hopes they will speak bluntly, but it does no good to join forces with cranks and quacks, magicians and madmen.
> (Glymour and Stalker 1983: 963)

or it can be pooh-poohed, as in a recent editorial in *The New York Times*:

> At least as a sign of popular discontent, the holistic movement deserves serious consideration. Doctors do rely too much on drugs. Proper nutrition was until recently neglected in medical education. Medical specialists do not always convey the impression that they are greatly inter-

ested in the whole organism. . . . To dismiss holistic medicine entirely would be an error. Much that is orthodox was
once heterodox: witness the initial opposition to Pasteur's
germ theory of disease and Lister's discovery of antisepsis.
Some holistic practices, like acupuncture, may find a niche
in orthodox practice. But many are set irredeemably outside
the tradition of western medicine. . . . Its emphasis on nutrition, exercise and preventive care is well placed. But with
the first twinge of sickness, holism should be quickly forgotten. And doctors who claim to practice it are, at best,
borrowing the holistic label.   (Wade 1983)

Other articles have gone to great lengths to show that whatever
could possibly be good in alternative medicine is already incorporated in scientific medicine, that only the irrational is left
out. Most alternatives to scientific medicine are reconstruc-
tions of older healing modalities that were practiced prior to the
ascendence of scientific medicine. There have been few new
"healing modes," only new jargon, old wine in new jugs. A new
modality of healing based on an alternative epistemology of
health is clearly needed, and may, in time, result. It may not
have any relation to any of the current alternative practices now
in vogue. It seems likely though that it will utilize some concepts upon which alternatives base themselves as articulated in
the remaining chapters of this volume.

References

Ackerknecht, E.H. (1968) *A Short History of Medicine*. New York:
    Ronald Press.
Berliner, H.S. (1973) The Origins of Health Insurance for the Aged.
    International Journal of Health Services 3(3): 465–74.
——(1975) A Larger Perspective on the Flexner Report. *International
    Journal of Health Services* 5(4): 573–92.
——(1977) *Philanthropic Foundations and Scientific Medi-
    cine*. Unpublished doctoral Thesis, Johns Hopkins University,
    Baltimore.
——(1983) Medical Modes of Production. In A. Treacher and P. Wright
    (eds) *The Social Construction of Medicine*. Edinburgh: University
    of Edinburgh Press.
Berliner, H.S. and Salmon, J.W. (1979) The New Realities of Health
    Policy. *Journal of Alternative Human Services* 5(2): 13–16.

Berliner, H.S. and Salmon, J.W. (1980) The Holistic Alternative to Scientific Medicine: History and Analysis. *International Journal of Health Services* 10(2): 133–47.

Bonner, T.N. (1963) *American Doctors and German Universities.* Lincoln: University of Nebraska Press.

Corner, G.W. (1965) *A History of the Rockefeller Institute.* New York: Rockefeller Institute Press.

Daniels, G.H. (1971) *Science in American Society: a Social History.* New York: Knopf.

Day, S. (1982) Is Obstetric Technology Depressing? *Radical Science Journal* 12: 17–45.

Duffy, J. (1979) *The Healers: A History of American Medicine.* Urbana: University of Illinois Press.

Eyer, J. (1975) Hypertension as a Disease of Modern Society. *International Journal of Health Services* 5(4): 539–58.

Flexner, A. (1910) *Report on Medical Education in the United States and Canada.* New York: Carnegie Foundation.

Frankfort, E. (1973) *Vaginal Politics.* New York: Bantam.

Gates, F.T. (1923) Civilization and Disease. Speech presented to the Board of Trustees, New York: Rockefeller Foundation Archives.

Glymour, C. and Stalker, D. (1983) Engineers, Cranks, Physicians, Magicians. *New England Journal of Medicine* 308(16): 960–63.

Grana, J. (1982) The Aged in America. *Health Affairs* 1(2): 103–09.

Illich, I. (1976) *Medical Nemesis.* New York: Pantheon.

Jefferies, M. (1983) The Over-Eighties in Britain: the Social Construction of Panic. *Journal of Public Health Policy* 4(3): 367–72.

Kaptchuk, T.J. (1983) *The Web that has no Weaver: Understanding Chinese Medicine.* New York: Congdon & Weed.

McKeown, T. (1971) A Historical Appraisal of the Medical Task. In G. McLachan and T. McKeown (eds) *Medical History and Medical Care.* Oxford: Oxford University Press.

McKinlay, J.B. and McKinlay, S.M. (1977) The Questionable Contribution of Medical Measures to the Decline in Mortality in the United States in the Twentieth Century. *Milbank Memorial Fund Quarterly Health and Society* 55: 405–28.

Powles, J. (1973) On the Limitations of Modern Medicine. *Science, Medicine and Man* 1(1): 1–30.

Relman, A. (1980) The New Medical-Industrial Complex. *New England Journal of Medicine* 303(17): 963–70.

Rosen, G. (1958) *A History of Public Health.* New York: MD Publications.

Rothstein, W.G. (1968) *American Physicians in the Nineteenth Century.* Baltimore: Johns Hopkins Press.

Salmon, J.W. (1975) The Health Maintenance Organization Strategy. *International Journal of Health Services* 5(4): 609–24.

——(1982) Competitive Health Strategies: Fighting for Your Health. *Health and Medicine* 1(2): 21–30.

Sheps, C.G. and Lewis, I.G. (1983) *The Sick Citadel*. Boston: Oelgelschlager, Gunn & Hain.

Shryock, R.H. (1936) *The Development of Modern Medicine*. Philadelphia: University of Pennsylvania Press.

Susser, M.W. and Watson, M. (1971) *Sociology in Medicine*. Oxford: Oxford University Press.

United States Department of Health and Human Services (1980) *Health USA–1980*. Washington, DC: Government Printing Office.

——(1981) *Working Paper on Long Term Care*. Washington, DC: Government Printing Office.

United States Office of Technology Assessment (1978) *Assessing the Effectiveness of Medical Technology*. Washington, DC: Government Printing Office.

Wade, N. (1983) The Hole in Holistic Medicine. *New York Times*, 30 April: A22.

Wartofsky, M. (1975) Organs, Organisms and Disease: Human Ontology and Medical Practice. In H.T. Engelhardt, Jr. and S.F. Spicker (eds) *Evaluation and Explanation in the Biomedical Sciences*. Boston: D. Reidel.

World Almanac (1904) *Mortality Statistics*. New York: World Almananc Co.

—— (1983) *Mortality Statistics*. New York: World Almanac Co.

Two

Homoeopathy

Harris L. Coulter

In many countries a growing minority of physicians is abandoning conventional therapeutics for the doctrines of homoeopathy – a system of practice first described two centuries ago by the German physician, Samuel Hahnemann (1755–1843). They have their own societies and periodicals, their own textbooks, their own medicinal drugs, pharmacies and manufacturers. They consider homoeopathy to be diametrically opposed to conventional medicine (which they call "allopathy" or "allopathic medicine"), and they are often licensed as a separate medical profession.

Homoeopaths treat every ailment to which flesh is heir – epidemic infections, traumas, chronic and degenerative diseases – indeed, all the sicknesses and disabilities which bring patients into physicians' offices. They compete with the latest discoveries of twentieth-century medical research and the latest products of twentieth-century medical education.

Allopathy is unable to explain this phenomenon. Recognizing legitimacy in a competing therapeutic system is psychologically and politically difficult. Hence, the usual response is to ignore these practitioners. Since the mid-nineteenth century no American medical journal has published an article describing homoeopathic research or therapeutic experience. Medical historians have ignored this school almost completely. In private conversations and public pronouncements organized allopathy behaves as if homoeopathy does not exist.

But this response can hardly be considered adequate, if only because homoeopathy has doggedly survived and, in recent years, entered a period of vigorous growth. It is likely to remain a feature of medicine for the foreseeable future. Some knowledge of its history and philosophy, its triumphs and its vicissitudes is a necessity. What is more, it will shed light on the dynamics of conventional medicine today and tomorrow.

History and development

The name "homoeopathy" (also spelled "homeopathy") was coined by Hahnemann from the Greek words, *homoios pathos*, meaning "similar sickness." It signifies that what makes sick can also make well, or, in other words, that the patient should be treated with the "similar" medicine (Hahnemann 1982: 26).

The concept of "similars" is mentioned in the Hippocratic Corpus and has figured ever since as a current in western medical speculation. But prior to Hahnemann its meaning was never clear (Coulter 1975: 206). In the Middle Ages "similarity" was interpreted to mean the supposed resemblance between the medicine's physical shape or color and the part of the patient's body, or the "disease," in which it was thought to act beneficially (also known as the "doctrine of signatures"), leading to such prescriptions as walnuts in brain diseases and red coral in hemorrhages. At other times it has had other acceptations.

Hahnemann had little patience with the doctrine of signatures, and in the 1790s he discovered a new interpretation of "similarity." Knowing that quinine was curative in malaria, he decided to ascertain its effects on a healthy person. He took a strong dose himself and soon started to exhibit the typical symptoms of malaria. He concluded that quinine acts curatively in this disease because of its capacity to elicit malarial symptoms in a healthy person (now called "cinchonism" or "quininism") (Coulter 1977: 361; *Gould's Medical Dictionary*: 322).

He proceeded to explore this phenomenon by testing common medicinal substances on himself, his family, and his friends, a process which he called *Pruefung* (meaning "test" or "trial") and which, in the Anglo-American homoeopathic tradition is known as "proving." It involved administering the substance in tiny doses over a period of weeks or months and observing the symptoms produced (Coulter 1977: 363). These were recorded and became the methodological basis of the emerging homoeopathic system.

The proving as an a priori technique for ascertaining the curative potential of a medicinal substance was a completely new idea in western medicine. Hahnemann developed it systematically, publishing the records of sixty-eight provings in his *Materia Medica Pura* (Hahnemann 1880). About 600 substances had been proved by the end of the nineteenth century, and today the homoeopathic materia medica contains the provings (some only partial) of about 1,500 medicinal substances from the animal, vegetable, and mineral worlds.

These data are set forth in three classics: Constantine Hering's *Guiding Symptoms of Our Materia Medica* (Hering 1879–1891), Timothy Field Allen's *Encyclopedia of Pure Materia Medica* (Allen 1874–1879), and James Tyler Kent's *Repertory of the Homoeopathic Materia Medica* (Kent 1961). While today the Allen *Encyclopedia* is primarily a reference work, the Hering and Kent compendia have been reprinted regularly and remain the indispensable guides to homoeopathic practice.

When treating a patient the homoeopathic physician first notes down his symptom-pattern and then compares it with the patterns from the provings. The medicine whose symptomatology in the provings is closest to that of the patient will be the "most similar" medicine (the "simillimum") and thus the one indicated. Mere superficial similarity between the two symptom-patterns is not sufficient. Only the medicine which is "most similar" will have a truly curative effect (Kent 1979: 201; Hahnemann 1982: 121, 135).

Hahnemann called the "law of similars" a law of nature, and this remains the opinion of his followers today (Coulter 1977: 362). The practice based upon this law is thus a true science, the "science of therapeutics," which explains why the principles of homoeopathy have not altered in any essential way since Hahnemann's day. While generations of practitioners have added new information to the existing body of data, homoeopathy's theoretical structure has never changed in any essential.

Allopathic critics often reproach it for allegedly failing to keep up with medical and scientific progress, for rejecting the therapeutic fashions which come and go with the decades (it has been remarked that the "half-life" of a medical fact is about five years). The only possible response is that a true science does not undergo unending revision. The laws of physics, mathematics, and chemistry are not altered in every generation. Why should this occur in medicine, and why should it be a sign of "progress?" That homoeopathy is methodologically stable should be taken as evidence of its scientific validity.

Of interest in this connection is the homoeopathic discovery that the folk medicines used in Europe and elsewhere since time immemorial often operated by the law of similars (Coulter 1973). This is true for colchicum in gout, camomile for the afterpains of birth, arnica for bruises and sprains, stramonium for certain types of mental illness, strychnine for muscular cramps and paralyses, and many others, some of which have made their way into mainstream medicine. When Hahnemann first set out to prove them, he found that they yielded symptoms identical with those of the ailments in which they had traditionally been employed (Hahnemann 1880). Mercurial preparations, used to treat syphilis since the late fifteenth century, have been found to yield the typical symptoms of syphilis (of course, in a very mild form) in the provings, explaining mercury's efficacy in this traditional application. Mention has already been made of quinine's homoeopathicity to malaria. These long-lived drug uses, like the longevity of homoeopathy itself, reflect dependence on the natural law of similars.

Homoeopathy came to the United States in 1825. Within two decades some of the prominent physicians of New York, Philadelphia, and Boston had accepted it, and in 1844 they founded the American Institute of Homoeopathy as the country's first national medical association (Coulter 1982: 124–26). Allopathy was seriously disturbed by these homoeopathic inroads and viewed establishment of the

Institute as a move to assert control over all American medical practice. Its reaction was to organize the American Medical Association in 1846. Homoeopathic physicians were not allowed as members, and professional contact between homoeopaths and allopaths was prohibited by the newly minted Code of Ethics (Coulter 1982: 179 ff).

Relations between the two branches of the medical profession in the United States remained intensely hostile until the early twentieth century when the gradual decline of homoeopathy made the question moot. During subsequent decades the imminent disappearance of homoeopathy was confidently predicted by leading allopathic physicians and officials of medical societies, but in the 1960s the movement took on new vitality and is today once again on an upward development curve. This revival, after a half-century of neglect and decline, has renewed interest in homoeopathy's therapeutic method and social history.

Some quite recent historical research has laid to rest one widespread misconception – that the homoeopathic doctrine was merely the brainchild of Samuel Hahnemann and had no doctrinal relationship to the general history of medicine in the west. It is now known that nearly all the homoeopathic ideas (the major exception being the proving) are deeply rooted in the western medical tradition and are in many instances found in the Hippocratic Corpus. Homoeopathy must be viewed as the modern expression of an ancient system of therapeutic practice.

In Greece and Rome this trend was represented by the Empirical School. After the Dark Ages it reemerged in the writings of the Swiss physician, Theophrastus Paracelsus (1490–1541) and was taken up subsequently by such less known figures as the Fleming, Jan Baptista Van Helmont (1578–1644), the Englishman, Thomas Sydenham (1642–1689), the German, Georg Ernst Stahl (1660–1734), and the Frenchman, Theophile Bordeu (1722–1776) (Coulter 1975, 1977).

The medical Empirics have always espoused a vitalist physiology, meaning by this that the living organism is capable of reacting protectively and purposefully to life's stresses and insults. Furthermore, they maintained, these reactions cannot be determined a priori but are always adapted to the nature of the stress. The living organism is subject to its own inherent rules and laws. Its actions cannot be predicted, even less "explained," in terms of relationships developed in other areas and disciplines. The only sources of knowledge of this unique living organism are the sense perception and experience of the skilled observer.

Opposition to this Empirical view in ancient times came from the Rationalist school (the ancestor of modern allopathy) which held that formal logic is a valid source of medical knowledge. The Empirics disputed this, holding that the discipline of logic could, as little as any other, predict the myriad purposive reactions of the living organism in health and disease.

In recent centuries Empiricism has questioned the relevance of physics and chemistry (biophysics, biochemistry) to medicine on the ground that the body's liquids and solids react differently *in vitro* than *in vivo*. These auxiliary sciences are incapable of envisaging the organism as a whole. Their rules are only partial and do not represent true observation and experience, which must be of the whole body. The physician treats the whole body, not some tiny part of it, and the source of this knowledge must be commensurate with its object. Only information obtained from experience with the whole body can provide guidance to treating the whole body. The patient's symptoms are what first strike the attention of the observing physician, and the Empiricists based their method on the precise notation and analysis of symptomatic knowledge. They rejected attempts to penetrate beneath the surface and elicit "mechanisms," holding that such knowledge was speculative and unreliable, not to be compared with the firmness and reliability of symptoms (Coulter 1975: 248, 270).

Empiricism was very concerned with the problem of reliability. Empiricists asked: "How can the physician be absolutely certain that his knowledge is accurate, in a matter as important as the preservation of life?" Knowledge becomes reliable when it is agreed to by all. When all can perceive, discuss, make comparisons, and draw conclusions, the resulting knowledge is reliable. Hence only the symptoms can be reliable, never internal processes and "mechanisms."

Hahnemann was aware of the Empirical tradition and spoke favorably of it. He accepted its challenge to achieve a scientific method in medicine based on sensory data alone. His discovery of the proving was a major step in this direction: a reliable technique for obtaining a priori knowledge of the curative powers of medicines through observing their effects in the healthy. The medicines were proved in living persons whose reactions, as perceived by themselves and by others constituted the description of the medicine's action. And this knowledge could be applied in the same way, by observing the patient's visible symptoms and comparing them with symptoms from the provings. The homoeopathic method based on the proving thus employed sensory data alone and needed no speculative conclusions about processes occurring inside the body beyond the reach of the senses. Of course, it relies on the hypothesis that the law of similars is scientifically accurate, i.e. scientific truth. If this hypothesis is correct, a science of therapeutics employing sensory data exclusively is available to the physician.

Homoeopathic principles and practice

Hahnemann laid down three principles of homoeopathic prescribing: (1) selection of the remedy in accordance with the law of similars; (2) the single remedy; and (3) the minimum dose (Hahnemann 1982: 121, 197, 202).

Selecting the remedy on the basis of the law of similars is, in principle, so straightforward that the uninformed might regard homoeopathy as a rather simple system of medicine. In fact, it is excessively difficult, and years of training are required to develop skill.

Making a thorough and accurate physical examination is one of the most difficult medical arts. And the homoeopath must ascertain the patient's mental state as well, since mental symptoms are often the most important. Much practice in observation, questioning, weighing, and analyzing is needed to penetrate to the essential in the patient's symptom picture.

For the merely "similar" remedy will have little, if any, effect. Only the "most similar", out of the 1,000 or 1,500 medicines available, will truly help the patient. But the symptom pictures of many medicines resemble one another. They all have headaches, diarrhoeas, stomach upsets, joint aches and pains, and the like. These same symptoms are also found in most patients, whatever the ailment or illness from which they may be suffering. How is the physician to distinguish patients and medicines from one another with sufficient precision to arrive infallibly at the "most similar?" (Hahnemann 1982: 121, 135).

The solution was to subdivide symptoms and classify them by order of importance. This issue had already been faced in the Empirical tradition. As early as the second or first centuries BC they had resolved that the more important symptoms were the ones encountered rarely – in few patients or in few "diseases." The less important were those encountered frequently – in many patients and many "diseases." The former they called the "peculiar" symptoms (Latin: *propria*), the latter the "common" symptoms (Latin: *communia*) (Coulter 1975: 250).

While clear enough in principle, however, in practice this procedure turned out to be fraught with methodological pitfalls. How can a symptom be defined in such a way as to mean the same to everyone? How are physicians to decide which symptoms occur more or less frequently than others? Books were written on this up into the nineteenth century, but no satisfactory answer was ever provided. For two millennia it remained a major stumbling-block of the Empirical method.

Hahnemann's proving lifted Empiricism over this obstacle and permitted a new and long-lasting formulation of the traditional doctrine. For it revealed that *medicines* also have their "common" and "peculiar" features. The former are the symptoms found in the provings of most or all medicines, while the latter are those associated with only one medicine, or a few. The homoeopaths found that the provings of nearly all medicines yield headaches, neuralgias, diarrhoeas, rheumatic aches and pains, and the like. But each medicine also possesses features found rarely, if at all, in the provings of other medicines.

For instance, the proving of *Sulphur* gives rise to heat in the extremities; the patient who needs this medicine will often sleep with his feet outside the bedcovers (Boericke 1976: 622). The medicine made from the poison of the bushmaster snake (*Lachesis*) is characterized by left-sidedness of all complaints (Nash 1913: 111; Boericke 1976: 390). The common dandelion (*Taraxacum*) has "loquacity and inclination to laughter" (Clarke 1925: III, 1370). *Spigelia* patients are "afraid of sharp and pointed things, pins, needles, etc." (Boericke 1976: 601).

Sodium chloride (*Natrium muriaticum*) patients are described as "depressed . . . consolation aggravates" (Nash 1913: 325). Thornapple (*Stramonium*) has "devout, earnest, beseeching, and ceaseless talking" (Boericke 1976: 612).

When the patient manifests this "strange, rare, or peculiar" symptom, the corresponding remedy will usually be indicated, even though the common symptoms of the remedy may not agree completely with those of the patient. Furthermore, homoeopathy possesses a technique for converting common symptoms into peculiar ones. If the patient complains of a "headache," the physician will not be satisfied but will ask for further specification. Where is the headache localized? In the forehead, the occiput, the crown, or the temples? What is the nature of the pain? Boring, stabbing, throbbing, burning, like a band around the head, etc.? Is it continuous or periodic, and, if the latter, at what time of the day or night does it come on? These same gradations and variations of common symptoms are also found in the provings, offering a precise method of refining common symptoms into peculiar ones (Hahnemann 1982: 85 ff).

The homoeopathic method thus permits individualization of treatment on the basis of a strict method applicable to all. It is a science of the individual patient. Or, in other words, it is oriented toward the patient's idiosyncrasy which is the key to his illness and also to his cure (Hahnemann 1982: 126).

This stress on "idiosyncrasy" brings us to the heart of the contrast between the homoeopathic therapeutic method and the method of "scientific medicine." It is discussed further in the following section.

Hahnemann's second rule, the "single remedy," specifies that the patient should not receive more than one remedy at a time. While the prescription may be changed during the course of treatment, the physician may not administer two or more remedies at the same time – Remedy A for a part of the patient's symptoms, Remedy B for another part, and so on (Hahnemann 1982: 197). This rule reinforces homoeopathy's concern with the patient's idiosyncrasy. The purpose of the prescription is not to eliminate one symptom or another. It is to match the idiosyncratic essence of the remedy with the idiosyncratic essence of the patient. The symptoms serve merely as guides. A contemporary medical dictionary defines "idiosyncrasy" as:

any special or peculiar characteristic or temperament by
which a person differs from other persons. A peculiarity of
constitution that makes an individual react differently from
most persons to drugs or other influences.

(*Gould's Medical Dictionary*: 651)

Thus the patient's idiosyncrasy is the undefinable essence that
distinguishes him from all others. In itself it is unknowable.
But homoeopathy defines it operationally, for idiosyncrasy is
revealed by the patient's peculiar symptoms, while these same
symptoms in the records of provings point to the medicine
which will act curatively. The physician does not know the
essence of the patient's idiosyncrasy, but he can cure the
patient's illness with the similar medicine.

It is obvious why he should prescribe only one remedy at a
time. If the physician takes his indications from a part of the
patient's symptoms, he will not pinpoint the patient's idiosyncrasy, and the medicine will not fit. This defect cannot be
compensated by prescribing another medicine which also
covers part of the patient's symptoms. Only the arrow which
hits the bullseye counts in homoeopathy, not those which
strike other parts of the target. The physician is seeking the
"most similar" remedy, not those which have some superficial
similarity with the patient's symptoms.

Hahnemann's third rule, the "minimum dose," advises the
physician not to administer more medicine than the patient
needs. All healing is from within, and the physician is
supposed to stimulate the self-healing power of the organism
with his remedy. He is not supposed to overpower the body
and compel it to move in one direction or another. The
organism always (except when moribund) possesses some self-
healing capacity; by his correct prescription the physician
starts it on the path to cure. For this the minimum dose will
always suffice (Hahnemann 1982: 128, 202). These minimum
doses, however, have often appeared so tiny as to be
nothing more than placebos and have thus been a source
of friction between homoeopathy and allopathy. Why do
homoeopaths employ these very small, "infinitesimal,"
doses?

Initially Hahnemann prescribed medicines in the normal
dose range for his times. But he found that the "similar"

medicine intensified and exacerbated the patient's symptoms during the process of cure. He thus experimented with smaller and smaller doses and found that the aggravation of symptoms was greatly reduced while the curative powers of medicines remained unaffected even at infinitesimally small doses. In time dose levels of one millionth of a grain became very common in homoeopathy, while the very largest doses employed seldom exceed one thousandth of a grain. A further development of the minimum-dose doctrine has been the discovery that with further dilution the medicines alter their sphere of activity from the physical to the emotional and intellectual (Coulter 1977: 400, 403).

To charges that these medicines are only placebos the homoeopaths respond that they have been employed for almost 200 years in infants, animals, and unconscious persons, where a psychosomatic component is excluded. Why, in any case, would persons making a living in the practice of medicine employ drugs devoid of activity? Nothing compels homoeopathic physicians to use these ''high'' dilutions, and they do on occasion employ medicines in ponderable doses and even tinctures. They could, indeed, employ these latter exclusively. The reason they do not, but also make use of the ''high'' dilutions, is that they are efficacious. If they had not been, they would long ago have been discarded.

The employment of controlled clinical trials to compare the relative therapeutic efficacy of homoeopathy and allopathy has generally been stymied by the methodological difficulties involved in comparing two such different approaches, but a recent trial involving homoeopathic and allopathic drugs in the treatment of rheumatoid arthritis demonstrated homoeopathy's superiority (Gibson *et al.* 1980).

Other quite recent research suggests that in the very ''high'' dilutions (beyond the Avogadro Limit) the molecular structure of the medicine is transferred to the medium (an 87 per cent hydroalcohol solution), so that the medium becomes the carrier of the medicine's informational content. Thus the medium is the message (Coulter 1982: 52 ff)!

How does homoeopathic practice differ from conventional medicine?

The difference, indeed, the gulf, between homoeopathic and allopathic theory and practice is best understood by returning to the question of the common and peculiar symptoms. Homoeopathic method is based on the peculiar features of patients, their idiosyncrasies, while the common features are relegated to subordinate status. Allopathic doctrine, on the contrary, relies on the common symptoms and ignores the idiosyncratic ones. The operational entities of "scientific medicine" are "diseases," and diseases are described and defined in terms of the common features of groups of patients considered to be suffering from the same "disease."

What greater difference could be imagined? Every allopathic physician knows that patients often react "idiosyncratically" to treatment, have "atypical" diagnoses, and, indeed, suffer from ailments which are not described in any medical text. It is estimated that about half of the patients seen in ordinary practice today do not have any definite diagnosis. But "scientific medicine" has no methodological space for the unusual, the peculiar, the idiosyncratic. They are regarded merely as disturbing features abrogating the biological laws which should normally apply. While, in practice, the allopathic physician is well advised to pay close attention to these idiosyncrasies, they are not allowed for in theory. They are excluded from methodological consideration.

Allopathic medical science is formulated by abstracting from these idiosyncrasies and assuming a uniform pathophysiological process occurring under the surface. The heterogeneous mass of diseased mankind is divided up into a series of uniform "diseases" defined by the common symptoms of those patients thought to be suffering from the given "disease."

Thus the material which is of greatest use in homoeopathy – the idiosyncratic features and reactions of the patients – has no methodological role in allopathy. And the disease names and categories which are so essential to allopathy are useless information to the homoeopath. He employs them only for the sake of convenience or to reassure the patient (who invariably wants to know what disease he is suffering from). No group of patients supposedly suffering from the same "disease" in fact responds in precisely the same way to treatment or is sick in precisely the same way. Response to a morbific influence is always determined by the patient's underlying idiosyncrasy. Hence this is the focus of the homoeopath's attention from the outset.

The medicines used in the two schools are entirely different. The allopathic physician generally prescribes on the principle of "contraries," using medicines which are thought to "oppose" or "neutralize" some pathological process within the body of the patient. This can be seen from the very names of many modern drugs: *blocking* agents, *anti*bacterials, *anti* hyperlipemics, histamine receptor *antagonists*, immuno*suppressives*, and the like. But many other medicines are used in allopathy, consciously or unconsciously, on the principle of similars. For instance, nitroglycerine was discovered as a remedy for angina pectoris by American homoeopaths in the mid nineteenth century on the basis of its proving. Today it is commonly used by allopathy for the same purpose even though its "mechanism of action" is said to be obscure. Vaccination and desensitization therapy for allergies are other examples of the application of similars in modern allopathy (Coulter 1973: 71).

The homoeopathic physician, of course employs medicines only on the basis of the provings and in line with the law of similars. Thus he uses a quite different assortment of medicines and rarely makes use of an allopathic one.

The contrast between allopathic "contraries" and homoeopathic "similars" has a corollary in the attitudes of the respective schools to the innate healing capacity of the organism. The homoeopath, who has confidence in the organism's healing powers, interprets the symptoms as signs of this healing effort. Thus they are, in most cases, beneficial phenomena indicating the path being taken by the organism in its curative effort. By administering the similar medicine he is helping to promote this very healing thrust of the organism. The allopath does not have the same confidence in the organism's self-healing powers. He does not interpret the symptoms as beneficial but as harmful phenomena, the signs of an underlying deterioration of the patient's health, the external manifestations of an internal disease cause. The contrary medicine is designed to counteract this pathological process, to suppress and eliminate the cause by suppressing and eliminating the symptoms. Allopathy has no systematic technique for aiding and abetting the curative response of the organism (Coulter 1981: 26 ff).

Expressed differently, the allopath attempts to place his own stamp on the body, compelling it to move in the direction which *the physician* decides is correct. The homoeopath subordinates himself to the curative impulse of *the organism*, administering remedies which support and aid this impulse. And he prescribes them singly, in the minimum dose, while allopathy gives large doses and mixes medicines. Since he interprets the patient's diseased state in terms of causal relations inside the body, the allopath feels justified in prescribing a medicine for each cause. Homoeopathy rejects polypharmacy because it regards illness as a unitary disturbance of the body's vitality.

Each of the three homoeopathic rules of practice is thus at odds with allopathic theory and practice. And since homoeopathy considers its method scientific, the allopathic method cannot, in its view, also be scientific. The allopathic definition of medical "science" is patterned on physics, whose laws are developed by observing events which occur millions of times in precisely the same way and thus yield their connections and relations with other events which also occur millions of times in the same way. But, since biological events never occur millions of times, or even hundreds of times, in precisely the same way, allopathy abstracts from the heterogeneity of mankind by ignoring idiosyncrasy and assuming a uniformity which is not really there. The true variability of biological events, which can be observed every day in the practice of medicine, is considered secondary to an assumed underlying pathophysiological process. The stamp placed by the patient's idiosyncrasy on this process is considered an ephemeral phenomenon devoid of significance for the derivation of medical "science."

Homoeopathy explicitly rejects this interpretation of medical science. The object of the physician's concern is the single patient in his uniqueness and individuality, not the patient as representative of some hypothesized disease process. Any medical science worthy of the name must be capable of analyzing the single patient and providing him with the treatment which his idiosyncrasy demands.

Homoeopathy was thus one of the first systems of "holistic" medicine. What is the "holism" of the patient if not his idiosyncrasy? Much of the current controversy over the correct definition of "holistic medicine" would be resolved by a general appreciation of this fact. Holism means the unique undefinable dimension of the individual that brings him into focus and distinguishes him from all others. "Holistic" medicine could as well be called "idiosyncratic" medicine (Coulter 1981: 102).

The conflict between homoeopathy and allopathy is between holistic and reductionist medicine. It is what historians of science call a "paradigm dispute," in which neither side can convince the other because the parties lack a common frame of reference (Kuhn 1970: 43 ff). Paradigm disputes are often resolved through political struggle. The relations between homoepathy and allopathy have always been marked by a high degree of political hostility – only moderated in the twentieth century because of homoeopathy's temporary decline. As homoeopathy grows stronger in the decades to come, the political antagonism will inevitably intensify.

The real issue between them, which is usually obscured by the atmospherics of the paradigm dispute, is the definition of "scientific medicine." Although the word, "scientific," has been monopolized for centuries by allopathy and its Rationalist predecessors, Empiricism has always contested this claim and considers its own method more truly scientific for the reasons given above. One more may be added.

A genuine science grows through gradual increments of knowledge and undergoes fundamental revision of its tenets only rarely, as what has been called by Kuhn the "paradigm shift." In this respect homoeopathy is closer to the scientific ideal than allopathy, since, while knowledge of new medicines has been added to the existing corpus, the principles themselves have not altered since Hahnemann's original formulation. They will doubtless remain unchanged for the foreseeable future.

Allopathy, on the contrary, is in continual change. And each new formulation of doctrine nullifies a large part of existing knowledge. Allopathic knowledge is not cumulative, and the therapeutics of one generation is unrecognizable to the next. Practices and procedures disappear for a time and then reemerge. The reasons for the incessant change of allopathic doctrine are outside the scope of this study, but the fact itself is patent. It is even made into a virtue, a sign of "progress" (Coulter 1981: 93 ff).

But to admit the inevitability of change is to recognize the unreliability of what exists, and the homoeopathic critique of allopathy is thus given unwitting support. Is allopathic doctrine condemned to twist and turn forever in the corridors of time? If so the knowledge will never be reliable.

However, allopathy will never be superseded by homoeopathy. Being a more time-consuming and intellectually demanding mode of practice, the latter is condemned to remain in the minority. A medical science which requires elucidation of the unique and peculiar features of each patient must demand more thought and care than one which need only ascertain the common symptoms to assign the patient to the appropriate diagnostic category. Homoeopathic physicians cannot see 30–40 patients per day, but 15–20 at the most. They cannot assign nurses or physician's assistants to perform diagnostic tests, since this is the area in which the physician's skill is most needed. Homoeopathy does not favor the mass production of medical services but preserves the intimate bond between physician and patient which was the hallmark of all medicine in an earlier age.

Current status of homoeopathy in the world

The most striking characteristic of modern homoeopathy is its extraordinary vitality. After passing through a lull from 1910 to the mid 1960s, it has once again become infused with energy and is today increasing its numbers and influence wherever it is practiced.

In the nineteenth century the United States was the world leader of homoeopathy, with 15,000 practitioners, fourteen medical schools, dozens of periodicals, and medical societies in every state and large city. Most states had separate licensing boards for homoeopathic physicians, and they enjoyed the same legal status and privileges as allopaths and eclectics.

One carryover from this period was enshrinement of the *Homoeopathic Pharmacopoeia of the United States* in the 1938

Food, Drug, and Cosmetic Act as the legal standard for prepara-
tion of homoeopathic medicines. The eighth edition of this
Pharmacopoeia was published in 1979.

The number of homoeopathic physicians in the United States
declined from a high of 15,000 in 1900 to a low of about 100 in
the late 1950s. Two whole generations were completely lost. In
the 1960s, however, as part of the pervasive discontent with the
country's social and political institutions, medical students
began seeking therapeutic alternatives, and many ultimately
came to homoeopathy. Today there are several hundred allo-
pathically trained physicians practicing homoeopathy exclusively as well as several thousand who use it occasionally, not
to mention the many nurses, osteopaths, chiropractors, veteri-
narians, clinical psychologists, and naturopathic practitioners
who also employ homoeopathy.

There are four or five manufacturers of homoeopathic preparation in the US who carry on a large export business in these
medicines.

A milestone in the development of American homoeopathy
was the passage, in 1980, of a homoeopathic licensing law in
Arizona – the first step to reestablishing the dual licensing
system of the past. A similar law was adopted by the Nevada
legislature in 1983.

But there are still too few physicians to meet the growing
demand, and self-prescribing by laypersons is an important
component of the modern picture. It is facilitated by the
accessibility of the homoeopathic literature to persons devoid of
formal medical training. The records of provings are accounts of
the aches and pains of ordinary people, and newcomers to this
discipline are delighted to find the descriptions of symptoms
given in non-technical language. What is more, the prescriber
does not have to justify his diagnosis by converting the patient's
description of his symptoms into some technically defined disease category. While the intrinsic difficulty of homoeopathic
prescribing should not be underestimated, no linguistic obstacles are placed in the way of the non-professional.

Lay practice is also facilitated by the non-prescription ("over
the counter") status of nearly all homoeopathic medicines in
the United States. A number of guides to lay practice have been
published since the first one saw the light of day in 1835 (Constantine Hering's *Domestic Physician* (1864) which was long-

lived like everything else in homoeopathy, with the thirty-third German language edition being published in Stuttgart in 1946). The best recent domestic guide is *Homoeopathic Medicine at Home* by Maesimond B. Panos and Jane Heimlich (1980).

In its stress on lay practice, homoeopathy is in step with recent recommendations by physicians and medical organizations that patients receive more instruction in self-care to reduce costs and relieve the burden on the structure of medical services. Homoeopathic medicines are rarely harmful to the patient when incorrectly prescribed, and this built-in safety factor reduces the inherent risks of self-prescribing.

England has had a strong homoeopathic movement since the early nineteenth century. In recent years its public acceptance has been furthered by the patronage of the Royal family. The Faculty of Homoeopathy Act adopted by Parliament in 1950 accorded official recognition to the London Faculty of Homoeopathy and empowered it to issue diplomas of competence. Homoeopathic treatment provided by a physician is reimbursable under the National Health Service. There are about 300 homoeopathic physicians in the United Kingdom, and their numbers are growing steadily. Courses for physicians are conducted by the Faculty of Homoeopathy.

Homoeopathic lay practice is also strong in England, which has no law similar to the American "medical practice act" prohibiting the practice of medicine except by physicians. Laypersons in England may legally establish practices, and many have done so. Several associations of lay practitioners exist, conduct courses of instruction, administer examinations, and compile registers of qualified practitioners.

The Republic of South Africa has taken a novel approach to lay practice by establishing the South African Homoeopathic Association to which every lay practitioner must belong. The Association establishes conditions for admission, conducts training programs, and maintains a registry of qualified practitioners.

The medical professions of nearly all the European countries have well established homoeopathic minorities: France, West Germany, Austria, Italy, Switzerland, Belgium, the Netherlands, and Greece all have programs and courses of instruction for physicians, some private and others at the state medical schools. The pharmacies customarily stock homoeopathic medicines, and in some countries special laws have been adopted extending legal protection to these products. The 1978 West German Drug Law, for instance, established a separate register for homoeopathic drugs, and the French pharmacopoeia also has a separate section for homoeopathic products.

Mexico is perhaps unique among western countries in possessing two homoeopathic medical schools, one private and one governmental. Homoeopathy is strong also in Argentina and Brazil and is practiced in most other countries of Central and South America.

It is popular in Eastern Europe, especially the Soviet Union, but reliable information on the numbers of practitioners and the availability of educational opportunities is difficult to obtain. Homoeopathic products are produced by the state pharmaceutical manufacturers.

Pakistan, Ceylon, and India have been particular bastions of homoeopathy in Asia since the doctrine was introduced there in the nineteenth century by the British. The Pakistan government extended official recognition to homoeopathy in 1965, the government of Ceylon (Sri Lanka) in 1970. But India is the country where it made the greatest impression, with 125 homoeopathic medical schools, 3,000 homoeopathic dispensaries, and 150 hospitals. About 5,700 students study it every year, and there are 30,000 registered practitioners as well as another 170,000 registered lay practitioners.

Thus, although homoeopathy is a minority form of medical practice in every country except India, everywhere it has a loyal and tenacious clientele, and the prospects are bright for its continuing growth (Coulter 1981: 15 ff).

Policy implications

The problem facing policy-makers is the public's ongoing disenchantment with conventional medicine. After decades of over-confidence in doctors, a thoroughly skeptical attitude now prevails. Patients resent the mass production style of allopathic practice which emerged after World War II, with its high volume prescribing of "broad-spectrum" drugs. They resent the physician's unwillingness to spend more than a few minutes of his time with them. They resent the mounting expense. And, finally, they resent the apparent inefficacy of many of the procedures employed, together with the certainty of dangerous, even lethal, "side effects."

Indeed, the similarity with the early nineteenth century is striking. In the 1820s and 1830s the medical profession lost the confidence of the public. All protective laws were struck from the books, and for sixty years there was free competition among the therapeutic persuasions. Doubtless this cycle will now repeat itself. Since history moves faster today, it may run its course in less than seventy years, but some decades of stand-off between allopathy and the general public may still be anticipated.

The shortcomings of conventional medicine are not easily remedied, as the present abuses are part and parcel of the whole socioeconomic structure of modern medical services. More than good will or benevolent intentions will be required to eliminate them. In the meantime such medical alternatives as homoeopathy will have unequalled opportunities.

The public authorities can react in three ways to this novel situation. Least satisfactory would be abandonment of homoeopathy to the mercies of the allopathic licensing boards which have demonstrated so little sympathy to medical alternatives in the past. They would inexorably tend to suppress this competitor under the guise of promoting "scientific medicine."

Policy-makers must realize that homoeopathy is a different paradigm. It is not an auxiliary to conventional medicine, not a "specialty" form of practice, not an offshoot of nutritional therapy or spiritualism (although it has been called all of these). It will not in time "merge" with allopathy, since the two doctrines are opposed on all points. Homoeopathic physicians may make occasional use of other modalities, but these are in no way part of homoeopathy itself, which is a rigorous method for individualizing treatment by following Hahnemann's three rules.

Like allopathy, homoeopathy's subject matter is the full range of human illnesses. Hence it deserves a position of equality, the same rights and privileges as its main competitor. The most appropriate course for the public authorities would be to reinstitute the dual licensing system of the past. This has already been done in Arizona (1980) and Nevada (1983). Their example will probably be followed by other states in the near future. A dual licensing system could also take into account the different educational requirements of homoeopathic practitioners.

A third possibility would be to abolish medical licensing altogether, a step which has been advocated by some economists as a radical cure for the apparently uncontrollable inflation of medical costs. Although this may appear revolutionary, it is the system which obtains in Great Britain. There the unlicensed practice of medicine is permitted by law, and it has not led to medical or social catastrophe.

The course followed will depend upon the political circumstances in each state and the nature of the political leadership available. While the process of abolishing or instituting medical licensing boards is beset with difficulties, it is a normal part of the American political tradition and the appropriate way to deal with emerging social needs.

The legislatures will not be embarking into the unknown if they give support to homoeopathy. Its record over the past two centuries is open to inspection. It is a stable doctrine whose future will be not unlike its past.

The beneficiaries of such legislative initiatives will not be homoeopathy alone, but all forms of therapeutics presently described as "holistic." Hence any legislative effort will have broad public backing. The outcome will be a reorientation of medical thinking as allopathy is compelled to take into account the achievements of its holistic competitors. Ultimately the public will benefit from a genuine choice among therapeutic alternatives.

References

Allen, T.F. (1874-1879) *Encyclopedia of Pure Materia Medica: a Record of the Positive Effects of Drugs Upon the Healthy Organism* (10 vols). Philadelphia: Boericke and Tafel.

Boericke, W. (1976) *Materia Medica With Repertory* Philadelphia: Boericke and Tafel.

Clarke, J.H. (1925) *A Dictionary of Practical Material Medica* (3 vols). London: The Homoeopathic Publishing Company.

Coulter, H.L. (1973) *Homoeopathic Influences in Nineteenth-Century Allopathic Therapeutics*. Washington, DC: American Institute of Homoeopathy.

——(1975) *Divided Legacy: A History of the Schism in Medical Thought*. (Vol. I) *The Patterns Emerge: Hippocrates to Paracelsus*. Washington, DC: Wehawken.

——(1977) *Divided Legacy: A History of the Schism in Medical Thought*. (Vol. II) *Progress and Regress: J.B. Van Helmont to Claude Bernard*. Washington DC: Wehawken.

——(1981) *Homoeopathic Science and Modern Medicine*. Richmond, California: North Atlantic Books.

——(1982) *Divided Legacy: A History of the Schism in Medical Thought*. (Vol. III) *The Conflict Between Homoeopathy and the American Medical Association*, 2nd edn. Richmond, California: North Atlantic Books.

Gibson, R.G., Gibson, S.L.M., MacNeill, A.D., Watson, W., and Buchanan, W. (1980) Homoeopathic Therapy in Rheumatoid Arthritis: Evaluation by Double-Blind Clinical Therapeutic Trial. *British Journal of Clinical Pharmacology* 9: 453–59.

Gould's Medical Dictionary (1945) 5th edn. Philadelphia: Blakiston.

Hahnemann, S. (1880) *Materia Medica Pura* (trans. R.E. Dudgeon and R. Hughes) (2 vols). Liverpool and London: Hahnemann Publishing House. Indian Edition (n.d.) published by Jain Publishing Co., New Delhi.

——(1982) *Organon of Medicine* (trans. from the 6th edn by J. Kunzli, A. Naude, and P. Pendleton). Los Angeles: J.B. Tarcher.

Hering, C. (1864) *The Domestic Physician*, 6th edn. New York: William Radde.

——(1879–1891) *The Guiding Symptoms of Our Materia Medica* (10 vols). Philadelphia: The American Homoeopathic Publishing Co.

Kent, J.T. (1961) *Repertory of the Homoeopathic Materia Medica*, 1st Indian edn. Calcutta: Hahnemann Publishing Co.

——(1979) *Lectures on Homoeopathic Philosophy*. Richmond, California: North Atlantic Books.

Kuhn, T.S. (1970) *The Structure of Scientific Revolutions*. Chicago: University of Chicago Press.

Nash, E.B. (1913) *Leaders in Homoeopathic Therapeutics*, 4th edn. Philadelphia: Boericke & Tafel.

Panos, M.B. and Heimlich, J. (1980) *Homoeopathic Medicine at Home*. Los Angeles: J.B. Tarcher.

Pharmacopoeia Convention of the American Institute of Homeopathy (1979) *The Homoeopathic Pharmacopoeia of the United States* (Vol. I), 8th edn. Falls Church, Virginia: American Institute of Homoeopathy.

Homoeopathic organizations offering programs of instruction

International Foundation for Homoeopathy
1141 NW Market Street
Seattle, Washington 98107   (206) 789 7327

National Center for Homoeopathy
1500 Massachusetts Avenue, NW
Washington, DC 20005   (202) 223 6182

Society for Empirical Medicine
4221 45th Street, NW
Washington, DC 20016   (202) 362 3185

Three

Chiropractic

Ronald Lee Caplan

Introduction

Spinal manipulation is a very old therapeutic practice. Healers of ancient times were experts in the anatomy and mechanics of the spine and believed in the pathogenic effects of spinal misalignments (Bach 1968). In one of his many books on healing, Hippocrates wrote "Look well to the spine, for many diseases have their origin in dislocations of the vertebral column" (Wilk 1976: 17–24; Langone 1982: 5–6). More recently, two major schools of spinal manipulation have developed (Inglis 1969: 15; Bourdillon 1973: 1–4). Osteopathy was founded in 1874 by Andrew Taylor Still and chiropractic in 1895 by Daniel David Palmer. Today, most osteopaths have adopted the pharmaceutical and surgical techniques of modern medicine, and have largely abandoned the teachings of Hippocrates and Still. Only chiropractic, as a licensed health profession, specializes in the manipulation of the spine for the preservation and restoration of health (Wardwell 1978: 6–17).

Origin and historical development of chiropractic

Daniel David Palmer, a magnetic healer in Davenport Iowa, was the founder and first practitioner of chiropractic. The first spine adjusted by Dr Palmer belonged to Harvey Lillard, a deaf janitor in Palmer's office building. One day in September 1895, Lillard told Palmer that while working in a stooped position, some seventeen years earlier, he "felt something give way in his back and immediately became deaf." Upon examination, Dr Palmer found that a vertebra had been "racked from its normal position" and reasoned that its realignment might correct the disorder. Palmer repositioned the protruding vertebra and soon the man's hearing was completely restored (Luce 1978: 12–13). Encouraged by this result, Palmer further investigated the relationship between vertebral displacements and human disease. His findings, formally published in 1910, became the theoretical basis for a new healing profession. Since the manipulations were performed manually, Palmer called his newly discovered technique chiropractic – from a combination of the two Greek words *cheir* and *practikas*, meaning "done by hand" (Wilk 1976: 26).

Ironically Dr Palmer died in 1913, the same year that the first state law licensing chiropractic was passed in Kansas. Over the next fifty years, under the leadership of Palmer's son, chiropractic became licensed in nearly every state. By the mid 1960s there were approximately 20,000 chiropractors in the United States, treating three million people a year and receiving a total annual gross income of over $300 million (Smith 1969: 17). Chiropractic also flourished in Canada and Europe as prominent medical physicians acknowledged its therapeutic value (Wilk 1976: 192–203). This growing popularity of chiropractic challenged orthodox medicine and represented unwanted competition. In England, the British Medical Association (BMA) responded by recognizing the art of spinal manipulation as a new and legitimate medical specialty called either manual or physical medicine. In the United States, the American Medical Association's response to the "threat of chiropractic" was quite different. In 1963, the AMA established a Committee on Quackery, the expressed aim of which was "the containment . . . and ultimately the elimination of chiropractic" (Trever 1972: 4). For over a decade, members of this committee harassed the chiropractic profession and propagandized against it. In addition, the AMA formally labelled chiropractic "an unscientific cult" and forbade its members from associating with or referring patients to doctors of chiropractic. In spite of these efforts, American chiropractic continued to advance during the 1970s. In 1973, Congress voted to include chiropractic coverage under Medicare. In 1974, with the passage of legislation in Mississippi, chiropractic had state licensing boards in all fifty states. Also in 1974, the US Commission of Education formally recognized the American Chiropractic Association as the accrediting agency for chiropractic education, thus making accredited colleges eligible for federal funds (Miller 1975: 713; 1981: 40). In 1976, chiropractors in three states filed federal and state lawsuits alleging that the AMA, the American Hospital Association (AHA) and an assortment of other medical associations violated antitrust laws in their concerted efforts to monopolize American health care. In 1979, the state of New York filed a similar lawsuit and the Federal Trade Commission began its own investigation of possible restraint of trade violations (Booth 1981: 70–72). Pressured by legal fees of $100,000 a month and the prospect of future lawsuits, the AMA, between 1978 and 1980, revised its code of ethics. The new regulations allowed members to voluntarily associate with any legally sanctioned health care professional including chiropractors, and officially ended the practice of referring to chiropractic as unscientific. In addition, the AHA for similar reasons, agreed to allow its member hospitals to grant access to licensed chiropractors for a limited and specified range of services (Culliton and Waterfall 1979: 467; see also Allen 1979: 133–39; "AMA Drops Year Old Ban" 1980: 15; "AMA Withdraws From LCCME" 1979: 17; "AMA's Treatment of Chiropractic" 1976; Relman 1979: 659). Bolstered by these successes, chiropractic continued to prosper and by the early 1980s represented the world's largest alternative healing profession (Vogl 1974: 77–81; Van 1977; Treaster 1978: 26).

The basic principles of chiropractic and its differences with conventional medicine

The human spine is a flexible column of twenty-four interlocking vertebrae of the central nervous system. This stem, called the spinal cord, branches out through openings between the vertebrae to monitor and control cellular activity in all parts of the body. According to chiropractic, a vertebra can move so as to impinge upon a nerve. This vertebral misalignment, called a "subluxation," causes the transmission of impaired impulses and can result in a wide variety of bodily disorders such as peptic ulcers, high blood pressure, diabetes, epilepsy, and even cancer. Chiropractic therapy involves the detection and correction of these subluxations. The latter is accomplished without the use of drugs or surgery through a series of manual manipulations of the spine called "adjustments." These adjustments are designed to restore the proper functioning of the nervous system, thereby allowing the body to heal itself. Furthermore, it is claimed that regular chiropractic care will help maintain the patient's health (Langone 1982: 16–27). In brief, central to the theory of chiropractic is the existence and pathogenic effects of the subluxation. All chiropractors believe subluxations exist, that they play an important role in the disease process, and that the human body would be a great deal healthier without them.

Chiropractic thus represents an approach to health and health care that is uniquely distinct from that of conventional medicine. Within the paradigm of chiropractic, disease, germ theory, and even chiropractic itself, are conceptualized very differently than within the medical paradigm (Kuhn 1970; Nofz 1978). In fact, most of the theoretical conflicts between medical doctors and chiropractors (in addition to the economic and political ones mentioned earlier) center around their different and at times contradictory definitions of one or more of these fundamental concepts. For instance, medical doctors tend to equate symptoms with disease and health with the absence of symptoms. Simply put, the onset of symptoms is seen as the start of the disease process and their disappearance as marking its end. Hence, the principal role of the physician is to diagnose or identify the patient's particular set of symptoms and through drug therapy and/or surgery seek their elimination.

In contrast, chiropractic does not make this equation. The appearance of symptoms and the onset of a disease are not regarded as simultaneous events. Instead, a body is said to be at "dis-ease" for some time, perhaps even years, before the situation so deteriorates that noticeable and/or debilitating symptoms appear. Broadly speaking, a chiropractor is less concerned with the pattern of symptoms than with their underlying cause – the subluxation – and the resulting improper transmission of nerve impulses. Moreover, the location of the vertebral displacement along the spine determines where in the body the symptoms may appear. According to chiropractic, by removing the subluxation the chiropractor allows the body to effect its own cures and symptoms (such as pain, nausea, and fever) then disappear. The drug and surgical therapies of the medical profession are often seen as undesirable as they are intended to alleviate symptoms while ignoring underlying causes. For chiropractic, as long as subluxations exist a body cannot function properly and hence is not in a state of optimum health. This is true regardless of the appearance or disappearance of symptoms.

A closely related dispute concerns the differing conceptualizations of the germ theory of disease. Within the medical paradigm, germs are understood to be the underlying cause of a variety of disorders – from simple infections to more deadly diseases such as typhoid and tetanus. For these illnesses, the appearance of germs of a sufficient density and type mark the beginning of a specific disease process and their reduction below that level marks the onset of recovery. In this sense, germs are like symptoms – they both appear at the beginning of the disease process and their disappearance signals its end. In these cases, the proper role of the physician is to prescribe the appropriate medicine, usually some form of antibiotic, to help reduce the germ population and restore health.

According to the medical profession, this particular understanding of germ theory has been "scientifically" proven and hence constitutes the basis of what has become known as "scientific medicine." All practitioners not subscribing to this view are by definition "unscientific" and have been derogatorily referred to as cultists and quacks. Chiropractors' claim that subluxations cause disease appears to clearly contradict the "scientifically proven" germ theory, and hence is seen as outright heresy (Dekruif 1926). Up until quite recently, this was the official position of the AMA regarding chiropractic.

When accused of "not believing in the germ theory" chiropractors emphatically assert that they are in complete agreement with a slightly different, but no less scientific, understanding of the germ theory (Kuxhaus 1969: 83-9). The role of germs in the disease process is reconceptualized within the chiropractic paradigm and the reformulated germ theory is completely consistent with the practice of chiropractic. Specifically, chiropractors maintain that germs are a necessary but not a sufficient condition for the onset of disease. For a disease process to develop and symptoms to occur, a "susceptible host" must also be present. According to chiropractic, the susceptibility of the host organism is key to understanding the pathogenicity of bacteria, viruses and other micro-organisms. In brief, an individual's predisposition to disease depends upon many factors, including heredity, environmental pathogens, poor nutrition, stress, and the presence of vertebral subluxations. The latter are believed to alter the nerve impulses to and from all parts of the body, thereby "causing lowered tissue resistance, a predisposing cause of disease" (Wilk 1976: 29-30). In such a suitable environment, a germ (which may normally be present) now multiplies and its presence in large numbers become part of the disease process – a symptom of the disease – instead of its cause (Verner, Weiant, and Watkins 1953; Thomas 1974: 75-80). Since the subluxation is a contributing cause, its removal is a prerequisite for health. However, most chiropractors believe that this conceptualization of the germ theory in no way precludes the possibility that a disease process can advance beyond the body's own curative capabilities and that drugs and/or surgery may be necessary for the patient's recovery. In such cases, most chiropractors refer their patients to medical physicians (Hildebrandt 1980: 25).

In spite of charges to the contrary, chiropractic does have a germ theory of disease. It is however a theory that differs from the one embraced by conventional medicine. But this difference clearly does not constitute sufficient grounds for dismissing it as "unscientific." It seems that the chiropractic paradigm is not so much "unscientific" as it is a *different* science.

A third somewhat less theoretical area of dispute concerns the proper role of chiropractic in the delivery of health care services. Some physicians, perhaps even a majority, insist that vertebral subluxations are an anatomical impossibility and label chiropractic a significant danger to the public's health (Ballantine 1972; Crelin 1973). Others in the medical profession view chiropractic as a highly specialized therapeutic practice best limited to the treatment of only obvious musculoskeletal conditions such as sciatica, low back pain and whiplash. By rejecting the claim that vertebral subluxations are in any way pathogenic, this definition greatly reduces the legitimate domain of chiropractic as well as the range of therapies it can offer (Brody 1975; Wardwell 1980). Needless to say, chiropractors reject both of these characterizations and insist they are "holistic healers" specializing in preventative care (Manber 1978: 58).

The current status of chiropractic

Unlike other therapies that have challenged orthodox medicine, chiropractic remains a thriving and distinct health care profession (Inglis 1969: 104). Because it represents a "unique and divergent paradigm of patient therapy," chiropractic operates and accredits its own schools, examines, board-certifies its own practitioners and maintains its own professional organizations.

Currently in the United States there are over 25,000 licensed chiropractors, about 80 per cent of whom are actively providing patient care. Although chiropractors can legally practice in all fifty states, the District of Columbia and Puerto Rico, their highest concentrations are found in the North Central and Pacific regions of the country. The South Central and New England states have the country's lowest chiropractor to population ratios (Brennan 1983). Approximately 40 per cent of the nation's chiropractors are in towns with populations under 25,000 people. Nearly all US chiropractors are white males whose average age is forty-five. Most of these practitioners operate a privately owned solo practice (Langone 1982: 47–9).

American chiropractic is ideologically divided into two major camps. The traditionalist and more conservative group, commonly referred to as the "straights," believe that the vertebral subluxation is the primary cause of nearly all disease and that proper chiropractic therapy consists only of spinal adjustments. The approximately 5,500 US chiropractors that support this definition of chiropractic generally belong to the International Chiropractors Association (ICA). The more liberal wing of the profession, known as "mixers," adopts a much broader view. While they agree that the vertebral subluxation can play an important role in the disease process, they refuse to limit their practice of chiropractic to only the correction of these misalignments. In addition to spinal adjustments, these practitioners also manipulate extremities, such as the knees, shoulders, and skull. Moreover, they may also employ ultrasound, electrical stimulation, vitamin therapy, special diets and nutritional supplements, vibrators, laboratory analysis, ultraviolet and infra-red light, muscle testing, whirlpool baths, bracing, and even acupuncture. In the US, chiropractors of this type number more than 17,000 and generally belong to the American Chiropractic Association (ACA) (Langone 1982: 28). Along with the fifty state societies, these two national associations constitute the organizational backbone of the profession. Although long standing hostilities remain, these two groups still are each other's closest ally (Gibbons 1979: 20).

There are presently sixteen four-year chiropractic colleges in the US graduating around 1,700 students a year. Although tuitions vary, the average cost per year is about $6,000. Applicants must have a high school diploma (or its equivalent) and have successfully completed two years of college. Like their medical school counterparts, chiropractic students must complete 4,000 hours of classroom and clinical work. With respect to the study of all the basic sciences, the two curriculums are quite similar. The major difference is that in place of surgery and pharmacology, the student of chiropractic studies spinal analysis and manipulation and nutrition (Simons 1980: 240; Langone 1982: 54–8). Before being able to practice their chosen profession, chiropractors must first pass national examinations administered by the National Board of Chiropractic Examiners and be certified by state licensing boards. However, unlike most medical doctors, chiropractors must participate in some form of postgraduate study in order for their license to be renewed.

Financially, American chiropractic fares quite well. Its services are covered by Medicare and Medicaid, nearly all Worker's Compensation programs and most health insurance plans. In 1978, total expenditures on chiropractic care were approximately $1.3 billion (Chiropractic Health Care 1980: XIII). Generally speaking, the typical chiropractor has 125 patient visits per week (compared to a medical doctor's 126), operates on a fee-for-service basis, and earns an average gross income of about $50,000 to $60,000 a year. In 1979, the national average cost of a chiropractic examination for a new patient, excluding X-rays and laboratory services, was $22.79 (Langone 1982: 47, 148). Chiropractors enjoy malpractice rates approximately fifty times less expensive than comparable medical coverage (Wilk 1976: 57).

Over the years, the public's use of chiropractic services has steadily increased. In 1978, nine to ten million Americans made about 130 million visits to chiropractic physicians (Treaster 1978: 26). Most chiropractic patients are female (56 per cent), between the ages of eighteen and sixty-four (78 per cent) and members of the lower middle income class. Many live in rural areas (Firman and Goldstein 1975: 640; Chiropractic Health Care 1980: XII). They suffer from a wide variety of conditions and most appear quite satisfied with the care they receive (Duffy 1979: 19–24). Chiropractic is clearly not, as some critics have charged, simply a "substitute" for less available medical care but is instead the *preferred* choice of millions of consumers (Yesalis *et al.* 1980: 415–17). In fact, it is the growing dissatisfaction with conventional medicine (embodied in the self-care and holistic health movements) that has substantially increased the public's demand for alternative therapies, including chiropractic. Chiropractors have long pointed out that well over one-half of all their patients are previously dissatisfied recipients of traditional medical care. One medical physician summarized the situation this way, "their [chiropractors'] successes are our failures." In brief, chiropractic in the US today is a well established and distinct health care profession with a well satisfied constituency of its own.

In the United Kingdom the situation is quite different. Most noticeably, there is no state oversight of chiropractic. Chiropractors are under no legal obligation to be registered or to prove professional competence. Simply put, anyone is allowed to call him or herself a chiropractor (*The British Chiropractic Handbook* 1983: 8–9). Under such arrangements determining the number of chiropractors is near impossible. However, according to the best estimates, there are approximately 3,000 practitioners of "massage and manipulation" in the UK and one chiropractor per 635,000 people in England and Wales. By way of comparison, the US has one chiropractor per 13,000 people (Shearer 1982; *The British Chiropractic Handbook* 1983: 11).

The British Chiropractors' Association (BCA), the profession's only national organization in the UK, was established in 1925 and currently has a membership of about 200 (*Register of Members* 1983). All members must have graduated from a recognized college and be willing to adhere to the Association's code of ethics. In an effort to upgrade the profession and protect the public, the BCA strongly recommends that only the chiropractic services of its members be employed. In addition, the BCA actively seeks the formal recognition of chiropractic as a legitimate healing profession fully sanctioned by the state.

The only approved British chiropractic college is the Anglo-European College of Chiropractic, founded in 1965 in Bournemouth. It was the first chiropractic college established outside North America and is supported by all the European chiropractic associations. The school's requirements take four years to complete and include an internship in an out-patient clinic, the passing of a comprehensive final examination administered by the European Board of Chiropractic Examiners, and the presentation of an original research project. Currently, there are about 150 students enrolled and nearly one-half of them are British nationals (*The British Chiropractic Handbook* 1983: 8; *Register of Members* 1983: 34).

As people in Britain become increasingly dissatisfied with conventional medicine, their demand for alternative therapies steadily rises (Mackenzie 1978; Inglis 1979, 1983). Because most of these therapies are excluded from the National Health Service (NHS), their growing popularity is largely confined to the upper income classes. A visit to one of these practitioners can cost the patient between £6 and £15 and only the affluent can readily afford to pay (Shearer 1982). There is however at least one indication that the popular support for chiropractic is somewhat more broad-based. In 1965, a group of satisfied patients founded The Chiropractic Advancement Association to help promote the theory and practice of chiropractic and obtain its acceptance as part of the NHS. Nationwide there are currently over 3,000 local affiliates (*The British Chiropractic Handbook* 1983: 10).

In brief, chiropractic in the UK is a much smaller and much

less developed health care profession than its American counterpart.

Future prospects: a critical appraisal

One obvious possibility is that existing arrangements will continue indefinitely. More specifically, chiropractic may remain a "marginal and deviant" profession and nothing occur to significantly change the scope of its practice. However, this prediction of long-run stability overlooks the fact that orthodox medicine, on both sides of the Atlantic, is currently in a state of crisis which is having a profound effect on all aspects of health care (Doyal 1979; Starr 1982). The crucial question it seems is not whether change will occur but what form it will take.

Another possible outcome is the cooptation of chiropractic techniques by conventional health care providers. In this scenario, manipulation of the spine would gain acceptance as a legitimate addition to the therapeutic arsenal of orthodox medicine. Increasing numbers of physicians and allied health professionals would, after relatively brief periods of instruction, perform spinal manipulations themselves. Already the armamentarium of physical therapists has expanded to provide numerous body therapies thought to be efficacious. To the extent that this practice became widespread, it would pose a serious threat to the economic well-being of the chiropractic profession.

As evidence mounts that spinal therapy can be an effective treatment for certain neuromusculoskeletal disorders, support for this particular pattern of development may indeed grow (Kane *et al.* 1974). However, the complete engulfment of chiropractic by conventional health care providers seems unlikely. In the US most physicians are untrained and largely misinformed regarding the procedures and clinical value of spinal adjustments. Moreover, American physicians have seemed quite unwilling to invest the time and effort necessary to learn alternative therapies. Adequately training such a reluctant group would, no doubt, prove to be very difficult and very expensive. The training of a sufficient number of physical therapists would also be a very costly undertaking. In Europe, a number of physicians do administer chiropractic type adjustments and these practices have been officially endorsed by the British Association of Manipulative Medicine. There the chances of a medical takeover of chiropractic are somewhat greater although they still remain quite small (Anderson 1981).

A third, and perhaps more likely, possibility is the eventual subordination of chiropractic by the medical community. This would entail the imposition of a strict set of limitations on the practice of chiropractic and the relegation of its practitioners to the status of "spinal mechanics" specializing in the treatment of neck and low-back pain (Thompson 1980; Hoehler, Tobis, and Buerger 1981). All causal relationships between subluxation and disease would be ignored and chiropractic would be stripped of its preventative dimension. In short, chiropractic would be subsumed within conventional medicine and lose its paradigmatic distinction. This approach is the current strategy of a small, but growing, segment of the medical profession ("Battle Line Between Medics" 1982; Serafini 1983).

For these health care reformers, this solution is considered desirable for at least three reasons. First, it employs tactics that have satisfactorily been used in the past against such former adversaries as osteopaths, dentists, and optometrists. Second, it would be less costly than coopting the techniques of chiropractic because it would employ the manipulative skills of already trained chiropractors and utilize already existing educational facilities. In short, it represents a more efficient allocation of resources. And finally, given the limited success of conventional medicine in satisfactorily diagnosing and treating most musculoskeltal conditions, the establishment of chiropractic as a manipulative therapy specializing in these disorders would provide physicians with a medically sanctioned outlet for these time consuming and troublesome patients (Fisk 1983; Firman, and Goldstein 1975: 641).

Chiropractic itself seems to be assisting in its own subjugation. The existence of chiropractic as a separate and distinct healing profession rests fundamentally upon the claim that a vertebral subluxation is a pathogenic condition and hence its elimination is health promoting. To their credit, the two American chiropractic associations in 1969 officially stated that the subluxation was not *the* cause of nearly all disease as D.D. Palmer had claimed. However, some chiropractors, particularly the so called "super-straights" have not yet completely disavowed this one-cause one-cure view of disease. The adoption of this extreme position by some over zealous practitioners damages the credibility of the entire profession. In the quest for greater acceptance and respectability, other chiropractors have accepted the limitations imposed by the medical community and have largely abandoned the defense of the subluxation altogether (Kruger 1981: 40; Moon 1981).

Perhaps even more harmful to the professional reputation of chiropractic, has been the absence of its *own body of scientific research* confirming and explaining the precise pathogenic nature of the subluxation and the health promoting qualities of its elimination. Instead, the profession has resorted to a much less rigorous and a much less convincing metaphysical and reductionist rationale for its existence. For example, efforts to defend and explain the therapeutic value of chiropractic by invoking such concepts as "nervous energy flows," "innate intelligence," and "the inherent recuperative powers of the body" without precise definitions or an explicit theoretical framework is little more than dogmatic metaphysics which convinces only those already convinced (Molthen 1968: 10; Gold 1970).

More recently, countless clinical studies have been generated that demonstrate, but in no way explain, the superiority of chiropractic in treating neck and back injuries (Potter 1977; Duffy 1978). The basic flaw of this approach is that nearly all of these studies reduce chiropractic to its least controversial application and then attempt to defend the entire mode of chiropractic care by demonstrating its efficacy in this single area. In order to establish itself as a separate and distinct paradigm of health care, chiropractic must "scientifically" verify its basic claim – that vertebral misalignments are pathogenic. In the absence of such evidence, demonstrating that chiropractic can effectively eliminate chronic low-back and neck pain serves only to reinforce the view that chiropractic should be limited to solely this function. In these ways chiropractors have undermined the establishment of chiropractic as a legitimate primary health care profession.

Although much of chiropractic research to date is seriously flawed, there do exist sufficient studies and an enormous amount of clinical evidence to strongly suggest the efficacy of chiropractic in treating a much wider range of human disorders, such as epilepsy, asthma, and diabetes. As one writer put it, "nine million patients can't all be wrong." (Treaster 1978: 26; see also Wight 1978; Weiskopf 1979). Consequently, chiropractic seems to represent an important and a much needed alternative to conventional medicine. If chiropractic works, but for as yet unknown reasons (as the evidence seems to suggest), then any one of the three scenarios outlined aboved would be therapeutically unsound, scientifically unjustifiable and clearly not in the best interests of the public. For these reasons, I propose a fourth possibility – one perhaps more difficult to achieve but representing a far more desirable outcome.

My proposal begins with the premise that chiropractic is a unique and potentially valuable paradigm of health care. Chiropractic is seen as being different from but not necessarily incompatible with conventional medicine. This approach stresses cooperation rather than competition between chiropractors and medical doctors. In a cooperative atmosphere of mutual respect and shared responsibility for the total health needs of the patient, the overall quality of health care could be significantly improved. This type of holistic approach is not without precedent. China perhaps offers the best example of modern western medicine existing alongside and cooperating with alternative health care modes to the great benefit of the patient (Horn 1969: 70–80; Sidel 1983: 209–39). On a much smaller scale, there are in the United States holistic health care centers which employ a multidisciplinary staff of doctors, ranging from medical doctors and psychologists to chiropractors and naturopaths and obtain quite favorable results (Buttram 1983). Establishing such centers at the national level is a more difficult but not an impossible task. In the UK, the inclusion of chiropractic into the National Health Service would be a comparable achievement (Barnard and Lee 1977). The remainder of this paper briefly examines some of the barriers that would need to be overcome and the chances of success.

Prospects for cooperation

At present the social environments in the US and the UK are not conducive to the establishment of cordial relations between the chiropractic and medical professions. Long-standing rivalries and deep-seated antagonisms are not easily put aside. While some progress has been made, many formidable obstacles remain. There are however some encouraging signs that these institutional barriers may one day be surmounted.

Perhaps the major stumbling block concerns the therapeutic efficacy of and "scientific" basis for chiropractic. Over the years, the chiropractic and medical communities have sponsored numerous studies attempting to examine and test the theoretical and therapeutic claims of chiropractic. Yet serious problems exist with *both* bodies of research. Most of the research generated within the medical paradigm is essentially of two types. It is either based on the a priori assumption that chiropractic is complete nonsense and thoroughly "unscientific," or that chiropractic is a marginal therapy, best limited to musculoskeletal disorders. This characterization of chiropractic by the medical community and the associated biases of the researchers themselves significantly influence the type of research undertaken – the methods employed and the conclusions reached. For example, much of this research utilizes cadavers or anaesthesia, neither of which are remotely involved in the practice of chiropractic (Crelin 1973; Webb 1977). Moreover, most medical researchers routinely conclude that any clinical success of chiropractic is due primarily to either the placebo effect or to the self-limiting nature of most diseases. However, since over one-half of the chiropractic clientele are dissatisfied medical patients, these conclusions seem highly suspect at best. More importantly, this body of research fails to adequately address two crucial chiropractic questions: are vertebral subluxations pathogenic and does their elimination promote health? Due to its inherent limitations, nearly all medical-based research of chiropractic is seriously flawed and contributes little if anything toward a meaningful evaluation of chiropractic as defined and practiced by contempory chiropractors. Instead, such research strengthens medical prejudices and only heightens hostilities between the two professions. In short, it is more of a hindrance than a help (Wilk 1980).

For chiropractic to be fairly evaluated it must be critically studied in its own terms – within its own paradigm. However, as noted earlier, too much chiropractic sponsored research has focused on the treatment of neck and low-back disorders instead of attempting to verify the very linchpin of chiropractic theory – the relationship between spinal misalignments and human disease. One chiropractor (Haldeman 1976) characterizes the situation this way: "Despite over 2,400 years of . . . (spinal adjustments) no group of health professionals has yet evolved which was willing to research the usefulness of this therapeutic procedure or to study the theories on which it is based." The danger is that in the absence of scientific verification chiropractors may dogmatically accept and defend the fundamentals of their profession while the medical community unjustifiably rejects them.

Over the last ten years some progress has been made. In 1970, for example, the University of Colorado in association with the National Institute of Health and the International Chiropractic Association launched a major research program designed to examine the relationship between vertebral subluxations and human pathology. By the mid 1970s, the spinal impingement of nerve roots was shown to be not only possible, but also capable of producing toxic protein substances (Simmons 1980: 238–40). In 1975, the National Institute of Neurologic and Communicative Disorders and Stroke (NINCDS), prompted by a Senate request for an "independent, unbiased study of the fundamentals of the chiropractic profession" sponsored a conference attended by 24 medical doctors, 7 osteopaths and 16 chiropractors to discuss and evaluate the scientific basis of spinal manipulative therapy. The participants concluded that the existing body of scientific evidence was inconclusive and called for more research (Radovsky 1975; Research Status 1975). However the fact that such an interprofessional discussion took place at all is an encouraging sign. Several years later, the government of New Zealand also released a study of chiropractic and its findings were quite supportive. However this investigative body – a three member commission consisting of a lawyer, a school headmistress, and a chemist – conducted no research of its own and based its conclusions solely on interviews and the cross examination of witnesses (Hocken 1980; Wilk 1980: 47). Although the scale of the study is quite impressive, in the course of twenty months the Commission compiled and evaluated over 1 million words of testimony, it does not represent a scientific assessment of the efficacy and theoretical underpinnings of the chiropractic paradigm. In short, this work, along with most other attempts to evaluate chiropractic, suffers from being too descriptive and too anecdotal in nature.

Compared to medical science, the science of chiropractic is still in its very early stages of development. Much to its credit the profession has quite recently sponsored some excellent paradigm-building research of its own. For example, last year the World Chiropractic Conference, an international group of chiropractors, medical physicians and scientists, met to discuss the scientific basis of chiropractic. Their findings were published in a most impressive collection of research papers (Mazzarelli 1982). Unfortunately, work of this kind is in rather short supply. It seems that most chiropractors, busily involved in their own private practices, fail to recognize the importance of this type of basic research and do not actively support it (Gibbons 1976). To help improve this situation, chiropractic colleges should significantly upgrade their research facilities and place greater emphasis on the teaching of research skills FACTS 1980: 57). Post doctoral programs should be instituted and students encouraged to participate. In brief, the specification and verification of the chiropractic paradigm should become the profession's top priority.

For major gains to be made the chiropractic community needs and should get outside assistance. The sophisticated research that is required calls for costly equipment, elaborate research techniques and a full-time staff of researchers. The chiropractic profession has neither the trained personnel nor the necessary financial means for such an extensive undertaking. Moreover, for this work to receive broad-based support it should be executed by an interdisciplinary group of scientists who publish their findings in highly respected medical journals. For chiropractic research to progress, public and private support will be needed (Collin 1980) and there are some encouraging signs that help may be forthcoming.

As federal deficits climb and economic recession lingers, the national government, in both the US and the UK, along with large corporations may eventually be willing to sponsor paradigm-building research for chiropractic as they did earlier in the century for conventional medicine (Brown 1979 and Doyal 1979). As part of an effort to reduce their spiralling medical bills, the public and private sectors may one day seek to establish alternative forms of health care such as chiropractic as safe, effective and less costly substitutes for traditional medicine. An additional and more direct incentive may be the heavy toll that back injuries exact within the sphere of production. In the US, nearly 20 per cent of all occupational injuries are related to the back and spine and on any given day 6.5 million people are incapacitated with some kind of back problem (Bergemann and Cichoke 1980; M.D. Jacobs 1980). In the UK, 88,000 people are off work each day with back pain and each year 26.4 million working days are lost – more than by strikes. Moreover, the annual cost to the UK in terms of lost production, medical treatment, and sickness benefits exceeds £1,000 million (*The British Chiropractic Handbook* 1983: 3). As clinical studies repeatedly demonstrate the superiority of chiropractic in the treatment of these disorders, the public and private sectors in both countries may, as part of their pro-competition strategy for health care reform (Salmon 1982), decide that the establishment of chiropractic as a viable alternative is in their own financial self-interest.

This outcome is by no means inevitable. Deepening federal budget cuts, a continuing economic crisis, and the certain opposition of the AMA and the BMA all represent formidable obstacles. Chiropractors have been legitimately challenged by the medical community to "demonstrate that their theories are sound, their diagnostic techniques accurate and their treatments effective" (Relman 1979: 660) and they should not be forced to lose by default.

Professional barriers

For a spirit of cooperation and reconciliation to emerge between the two professions, attitudes and actions on both sides must change. Members of the medical establishment must be willing to acknowledge the limits and inconsistencies of their own science as well as the possible existence of other worthwhile paradigms of health care. Specifically, the medical profession would need to realize that it *never* had a monopoly on medical truth and that *differing* viewpoints are not necessarily "wrong" or "unscientific." This would be in sharp contrast to the current situation where "modern medical principles have turned from a theory to a dogma and those who wonder what has been left behind are branded heretics" (Fulder 1980: 43–4). Arrogance and intolerance are attitudes that die neither quickly nor easily. For example, the AMA still stubbornly defines chiropractic as a practice based "upon the theory that all disease is caused by misalignments of spinal vertebrae and can be cured by manual manipulation and adjustment of the spine" (Burkhart *et al.* 1982: 105) in spite of the fact that both the ICA and the ACA have long ago disavowed any belief in a single cause or cure of disease (Savage 1980). Moreover, the AMA continues to insist that "no scientific evidence [exists] to support spinal manipulation and adjustment as appropriate treatment for human ailments . . ." (Burkhart *et al.* 1982: 105) despite the fact that such evidence does exist and is in fact growing. And finally, the AMA continues to warn the public of the dangers of chiropractic care even though the incidence of iatrogenic illness associated with chiropractic care appears to be negligible compared to that of conventional medicine (Hosek *et al.* 1981). Changing this hostility into an atmosphere of co-operation between the two professions will be difficult but not impossible.

According to Wardwell (1976), accommodation between "irregulars," such as osteopaths and more recently midwives, and orthodox medicine largely depends upon (1) the degree of perceived compatibility between the two groups' medical theories and therapeutics; (2) the potential for collegiality and mutual respect between the practitioners; and (3) perhaps most importantly, how willing the unorthodox practitioners are to subordinate themselves to medical supervision and control. With regard to the first there have been some encouraging developments. For example, as noted earlier, preliminary research indicates that spinal misalignments can cause the production of toxic substances. If these toxic substances can be shown to impair the body's natural immune system thereby increasing the individual's susceptibility to germs and viruses, then a major theoretical disagreement between chiropractors and the medical proponents of the germ theory could be resolved (Capra 1983: 128–30). Moreover if other pathogenic effects of the subluxation can be demonstrated, and it seems that they can, than a more complete reconciliation between the *two different paradigms* could also be accomplished. As iatrogenic disease continues at near epidemic proportions and alternative health care flourishes, as the very fundamentals of medical science are called into question and medical treatment for most chronic diseases remains largely ineffective, as the human body proves to be infinitely more complex than previously imagined and prevailing views of disease and health seem increasingly inappropriate, the medical establishment may become a bit less resistant to such developments (Epstein 1979; Capra 1983; Sidel and Sidel 1983).

With respect to the prospects for greater collegiality, there are some encouraging signs that long-standing barriers are at least beginning to crumble. In some instances by choice, but more often as a result of judicial action, a small but increasing number of chiropractors and medical doctors practice together in hospitals and offices, interact as members of state medical review boards and in other official capacities, such as county coroners and medical examiners, and socialize at professional meetings and conferences (P. Jacobs 1980). As these encounters become more frequent and a dialogue is established, especially among the professions' younger members, traditional hostilities may gradually disappear. One indication of a lessening of tensions is the steadily rising rates of referral between the two professions. According to a recent survey, nearly all chiropractors (96 per cent) regularly refer patients to medical doctors and 57 per cent of the chiropractic community can include among its patients the spouses and children of medical physicians (Brennan 1981).

The third major obstacle to improved relations, and one that will not be easily resolved, is medicine's insistence upon chiropractic subservience. Nearly every chiropractor rejects this para-professional status and adamantly opposes any attempt to reduce chiropractic to a sub-medical specialty limited to only the treatment of musculoskeletal disorders. Based on the experience of the osteopath, most chiropractors are convinced that acquiescence would inevitably lead to the demise of the chiropractic paradigm and they are probably correct. Furthermore, enough clinical evidence exists to strongly indicate that this outcome would be both unwarranted as well as unwise. Therefore, the medical profession should abandon its monopolistic schemes and stop harassing the chiropractic profession with unreasonable demands for dominance. Yet increasingly scarce health care dollars and growing competition among the health care professions greatly reduce the likelihood of this occurring in the near future (Relman 1983). Significant progress on other fronts and an improved economic outlook will undoubtedly be prerequisites for the surmounting of this particular barrier.

The eventual establishment of a partnership based on mutual respect and cooperation between chiropractors and medical doctors will also require a great deal of effort and good will on the part of the chiropractic community. Here too there are some encouraging signs. The determination of most chiropractors to survive as a separate and distinct health care profession is admirable, however mere survival is not enough. Chiropractic must precisely specify and develop its own *science* within its own clearly defined *paradigm* of health care. The emergence of a single scientific explanation and verification of chiropractic would greatly enhance the profession's prestige and credibility. It would, for instance, help in obtaining outside funding for research. The medical profession has already achieved this degree of unity and chiropractors should strive to do the same. As noted earlier, paradigm-building research is underway and though some chiropractors may resist or even defect this work should proceed without delay.

For relations to significantly improve between the two professions the long-standing feud concerning the diagnostic skills of the chiropractor will need to be resolved. Medical physicians repeatedly charge that because chiropractors are inadequately trained as diagnosticians they are unfit to be primary care physicians (Packo and Shaw 1980). Although these allegations are frequently exaggerated, they are to a degree justified. In the area of diagnostics chiropractic training is somewhat weak. Except for the Spears Chiropractic Hospital in Denver, no other facility in the US offers a residency program to chiropractic students (Luce 1978). Instead, most students obtain their diagnostic training in relatively small clinics where the number of patients seen and the diversity of disorders observed is rather limited. Consequently, the clinical instruction received tends to be more pedantic than practical and results in a fair amount of on the job training. This situation no doubt helps to explain the relatively small, yet not insignificant, number of chiropractic misdiagnoses of serious medical conditions resulting in the injury or death of the patient (Livingston 1971; Modde 1979; Gatterman 1981). While it is true that the number of malpractice suits against chiropractors is quite small compared to medical physicians, the frequency of these suits is increasing at an alarming rate (Jahn 1980). The lack of hospital-based training may be a contributing factor. At least, one chiropractor (Williams 1980) believes that it is and predicts that ''as long as chiropractors are denied access to diagnostic testing and laboratory procedures and equipment, and must rely on noninvasive testing and limited types of X-ray, there will be problems.''

While already serious, these problems could be getting worse. As the cost and sophistication of diagnostic equipment rises and institutional facilities such as hospitals become the only ones financially able to acquire and utilize this equipment, the diagnostic capabilities of the chiropractor may become increasingly inferior to those of hospital-trained physicians. This growing discrepancy could have a devastating effect on the chiropractic profession and on its relationship with the medical community. For these reasons, chiropractors should acknowledge the problem, recognize the potential dangers to their patients and their profession, and continue their drive to gain access to hospitals and hospital-based equipment.

As noted earlier, some progress has been made. Pressured by mounting lawsuits, the American Hospital Association has recently agreed to no longer censure a member hospital should it decide to open its facility to chiropractors. Nevertheless few US hospitals have, thus far, chosen to do so and most remain staunchly opposed. However, this resistance may be eroding. For example, as the relative cost-effectiveness of chiropractic in the treatment of various disorders is repeatedly demonstrated, a growing number of hospital administrators, increasingly concerned about profit margins and shrinking reimbursement payments, may decide to provide chiropractic care within their institutions for purely economic reasons (May and Henderson 1983). In this way the chiropractic community may eventually gain some powerful allies and gradually be accorded hospital access. Ideally departments of chiropractic would be established to provide chiropractic care to any hospital patient who might benefit from it. This approach would be far more desirable than the granting of admitting privileges to individual chiropractors and the limiting of chiropractic care to their patients only.

Although admittance of any kind into an existing hospital system promises to be a long and arduous ordeal, chiropractors should persevere and resist the temptation to develop a separate network of "chiropractic hospitals." A fully integrated hospital system would have several advantages. First, by avoiding costly duplication of equipment and facilities, it represents a much more efficient allocation of resources. Second, patients would be better served if they could receive both chiropractic and conventional health care within the same facility. And finally, by having chiropractors practice alongside of medical doctors, nurses, and a wide variety of other conventional health care personnel, age-old prejudices and mistrust may eventually give way to new-found friendships. For an atmosphere of cooperation and mutual respect to exist between the two health care professions, the biases and resistance of all concerned will need to be overcome. The likelihood of this would be greatly reduced if chiropractors became isolated in health care facilities of their own.

In order for the two professions to work together, either inside or outside of a hospital setting, chiropractors must demonstrate a genuine willingness and desire to cooperate with the medical community. A relatively small but quite vocal group within the chiropractic profession – the so-called "superstraights" – possess neither of these qualities and generally oppose any movement toward accommodation (Wardwell 1980: 689). Fortunately, they represent a disavowed minority. As long as the chiropractic profession itself is seriously divided on this, or any other major issue, the likelihood of reconciliation with the medical establishment is greatly reduced. Such internal divisions and disagreements weaken the profession from within, give ammunition to its opponents, and represent significant obstacles to progress. Chiropractors should take a lesson from medical history, resolve their differences and gain strength through unity. It is encouraging to see the "straight vs mixer" distinction become increasingly blurred and the extremists limited in number (Haldeman 1980). The eventual emergence of a single national chiropractic association in the US, financially and politically stronger than either of the two now in existence, would be a most encouraging development. In the meantime, improved relations and continued joint efforts on the political and research fronts are welcome steps in this direction.

Popular support

Traditionally, consumers have placed great faith in the value of drugs and the wisdom of medical doctors. However, by the early 1970s, people had been shocked by the possible side effects of some drugs and the inherent dangers of even the most routine medical procedures (Gerber 1971; Kennedy 1972). This growing disillusionment with orthodox medicine soon gave rise to two major reform movements – the self-care movement and the holistic health care movement. In both the US and the UK, these movements have contributed to the rising demand for alternative health care, including chiropractic (Inglis 1969, 1983; Mackenzie 1978; FACTS 1980: 77–90). Proponents of self-care have repeatedly stressed the limitations, the potential hazards, and the excessive costs of conventional medical care and advocate instead increased consumer reliance on self-care techniques (Fuchs 1974; Illich 1976; Levin 1976). These health care reformers have helped to convince millions of people that the public's uncritical acceptance of prevailing medical practice must end and that alternative care can be cheaper, more effective and safer (Caplan 1980; Salmon 1982). These changing attitudes indirectly encourage the public's use of chiropractic services (Inglis 1979). For example, as consumers become increasingly concerned about adverse drug reactions and unnecessary surgeries, chiropractic, a health care approach that employs neither of these therapies, seems particularly attractive. In this way, the success of the self-care movement is at least partly responsible for the growing popularity of chiropractic.

Advocates of holistic health care are also extremely critical of traditional medicine but unlike their self-care counterparts recommend the *purchase* of alternative forms of health care based upon a "superior understanding" of the human organism, its diseases and its optimum levels of health (Berliner and Salmon 1979, 1980). Specifically, the holistic movement defines health as a harmonious interaction among and between the external social environment and the internal human environment, consisting of the mind, the body and the spirit (Gordon, Hastings, and Fadiman 1981). Illness is seen as a result of an individual's inability to adequately adapt to these ever changing conditions. The holistic healer seeks the elimination of pathogens in both environments along with the improved adaptive capabilities of the total human organism (Pelletier 1979; Sobel 1979). This view of health and health care, with its emphasis on the prevention instead of the cure of disease, is extremely compatible with and supportive of, the theory and practice of chiropractic (Sullivan 1981). Consequently, chiropractic is usually included in the list of recommended alternatives which in turn directly enhances its legitimacy and popular appeal.

Without widespread popular support chiropractic has less chance of ever establishing itself as a paradigm of health care equal to, but distinct from, traditional medicine. The profession should not forget that the public represents its most important ally and do all that it can to promote consumer confidence and increase consumer demand. For example, in a move designed to broaden its base of support, the profession should more actively recruit blacks, Hispanics, and women to join its ranks. At present, nearly all chiropractors are white males. However, the racial and sex composition of the profession appears to be changing and the profession would be wise to encourage this trend (FACTS 1980: 98; Langone 1982: 47).

Chiropractors should also undertake a large-scale educational campaign to help counter over two decades of propaganda against them. In an attempt to debunk commonly held myths, the campaign should (1) define chiropractic as a unique paradigm of health care comparable to conventional medicine; (2) stress the preventative aspect of chiropractic and clearly explain the inappropriateness of limiting it to the treatment of only musculoskeletal disorders; (3) point out the error of abandoning the entire chiropractic paradigm if one of its practitioners proves unsatisfactory; and (4) continually inform the public of the latest scientific research regarding chiropractic. The degree to which the public is convinced of, or at least familiar with, the chiropractic viewpoint on these key issues will be a critical factor in governing the future course of the profession.

At a time when most patients do not pay their own medical bills the importance of gaining approval from third party payers, especially the federal government in the US, should not be underestimated. "If the present trend towards payment by third party payers continues, the time will come when the professional whose services are labeled worthless by the third party payer will face financial ruin" (Bachop 1980). Given this situation, the chiropractic profession should ascertain the criteria by which therapies are judged and do all that it can to qualify. Specifically, the profession should (1) establish a national definition of chiropractic so that terms such as "medical necessity" and "appropriate therapeutic care" have a precise and standardized legal definition with regard to the practice of chiropractic (Wiehe 1980); (2) conduct controlled clinical trials to demonstrate the efficacy of chiropractic care (Bachop 1980); (3) pursue basic scientific research; (4) seek to expand the rather narrow range of services currently covered to include "maintenance" or preventative care (Wardwell 1979; Mitchell 1980); and (5) substantially improve and intensify political lobbying efforts especially at the state and local level (Federal Legislation 1980; O'Bryon 1981; Booth 1981). In this way, chiropractors can help to ensure that their paradigm of health care is deemed worthy of reimbursement thereby bolstering the public's demand for it. Securing sufficient and stable funding sources is absolutely crucial to the long-run survival of chiropractic. Some analysts (Silver 1980) appear quite optimistic: "The policy issue will be, not whether chiropractic should be reimbursable, but under what conditions." However in an atmosphere of rising health care costs, prolonged recession, medical care cutbacks and mounting federal deficits the chiropractic community should be neither overly confident nor complacent (Arvidson 1981). In other words, the profession should remain vigilant and work toward the establishment of chiropractic as a complementary part of modern health care.

Conclusion

There is little doubt that the services of a competent chiropractor offer considerable therapeutic value (Silver 1980: 349). To the great dismay of some, chiropractic is not likely to disappear (Inglis 1979). However, chiropractors need to learn from the experience of the osteopaths (and more recently the midwives) and not allow themselves to be coopted by conventional medicine. The chiropractic profession should establish itself as a legitimate paradigm of health care distinct from but compatible with, traditional therapy. Anything less would probably result in its subordination to the medical community. If this was to occur chiropractors *per se* would still exist but their paradigm of health care, and perhaps even their professional stature, would not.

The actual outcome will be socially determined; it will be the product of complex interactions among and between economic, political and cultural factors. For example, the relative price of chiropractic care, the actions of government and the preferences of consumers will all have determining effects. Although the call for more scientific research should be heeded, science alone will not be the decisive factor. It should not be forgotten that chiropractic and modern medicine represent two different health care paradigms, each with its own science. Just getting the two sides to agree on the definitions of science and scientific research will itself be a major accomplishment.

Finally, it should be reiterated that there is cause for optimism. Barriers between the two professions appear to be slowly crumbling and a more favorable atmosphere of cooperation and mutual respect may be emerging. In some countries such as West Germany and parts of Canada these conditions already exist (Buttram 1983: 35). Various types of practitioners, such as medical doctors, chiropractors, and naturopaths, cooperating together represents a new division of labor within the health care industry – one that may be of tremendous benefit to the respective professions as well as to the public. Such an integrated or more holistic approach to health care would be well worth the efforts to attain it.

References

Allen, R.W. (1979) Medicine vs. Chiropractic: Our Leaders Let All of Us Down. *Medical Economics* 17 September: 133–39.

AMA Drops Years' Old Ban Against Chiropractic Profession (1980) *The Digest of Chiropractic Economics* (September/October): 15.

AMA Withdraws From LCCME, Modifies Stand on Chiropractors as Delegates Meet in Chicago (1979) *Hospitals* 16 August: 17.

AMA's Treatment of Chiropractic: A Case of Malpractice (1976) *Caveat Emptor* 6(4).

Anderson, R.T. (1981) Medicine, Chiropractic and Caste. *Anthropological Quarterly* 544: 157–65.

Arvidson, G. (1981) DC's Prone to "Sleeping Sickness": Leadership Seeks to Alert Members. *American Journal of Public Health* 18(10): 22–3.

Bach, M. (1968) *The Chiropractic Story*. Georgia: Si-Nel Publishing.

Bachop, W.E. (1980) Controlled Clinical Trials, Third Party Payers, and the Fate of the Chiropractor. *Journal of Manipulative and Physiological Therapeutics* 3(2): 93–6.

Ballantine, T. Jr, (1972) Will the Delivery of Health Care be Improved by the Use of Chiropractic Services? *The New England Journal of Medicine* 286(5): 237–41.

Barnard, K. and Lee, K. (1977) *Conflicts in the National Health Service*. London: Croom Helm.

Battle Line Between Medics and Chiropractors Drawn (1982) *The Digest of Chiropractic Economics* November 124.

Bergemann, B. and Cichoke, A. (1980) Cost Effectiveness of Medical vs. Chiropractic Treatment of Low-Back Injuries. *Journal of Manipulative and Physiological Therapeutics* 3(3): 143–47.

Berliner, H. and Salmon, J.W. (1979) The Holistic Health Movement and Scientific Medicine: The Naked and the Dead. *Socialist Review* 9(1): 131–52.

Berliner, H. and Salmon, J.W. (1980) The Holistic Alternative to Scientific Medicine: History and Analysis. *International Journal of Health Services* 10(1): 133–47.

——(1980) Health Policy Implications of the Holistic Health Movement. *Journal of Health Politics, Policy and Law* 5(3): 535–53.

Booth, W.S. (1981) Chicago Anti-Trust Trial. *ACA Journal of Chiropractic* 18(3): 70–2.

——(1981) Recent Legal Decisions Affecting Chiropractic. *The ACA Journal of Chiropractic* 18(3): 33–4.

Bourdillon, J.F. (1973) *Spinal Manipulation*. London: William Heinemann Medical Books: 1–4.

Brennan, M.J. (1981) Survey Results. *ACA Journal of Chiropractic* 18(4): 27.

——(1983) A Comparison of DCs and MDs. *ACA Journal of Chiropractic*, March: 32–5.

The British Chiropractic Handbook (1983) A pamphlet produced by the British Chiropractors' Association and the Chiropractic Advancement Association.

Brody, J.E. (1975) Chiropractic, Long Ignored as "Unscientific", Now is Increasingly Scrutinized by Health Specialists. *New York Times* 1 October.

Brown, E.R. (1979) *Rockefeller Medicine Men: Medicine and Capitalism in America*. Berkeley: University of California Press.

Burkhart, J.H., Sherman, S.R., Dobbin, B.A., Dickey, N., and Chisholm, W.S. (1982) *Current Opinions of the Judicial Council of the American Medical Association*. Chicago: AMA.

Buttram, H.E. (1983) Medical–Chiropractic–Naturopathic–Psychological Professional Relationships: A Model. *Journal of the International Academy of Preventive Medicine* 8(2): 33–5.

Caplan, R.L. (1980) Pasteurized Patients and Profits: The Changing Nature of Self-Care in American Medicine. PhD dissertation, University of Massachusetts.

Capra, F. (1983) *The Turning Point*. New York: Bantam Books.

Collin, H.B. (1980) Research in Chiropractic. *Journal of Manipulative and Physiological Therapeutics* 3(1): 37–40.

Crelin, E.S. (1973) A Scientific Test of the Chiropractic Theory. *American Scientist* 61: 574–80.

Culliton, B.J. and Waterfall, W.K. (1979) Chiropractors and the AMA. *British Medical Journal* 1(6166): 467.

Day, W.S. and Suh, C.H. (1973) Congressional Testimony for Chiropractic Research Grant. *International Review of Chiropractic*, October: 16F.

DeKruif, P. (1926) *Microbe Hunters*. New York: Harcourt, Brace.

Doyal, L. (1979) *The Political Economy of Health*. London: Pluto Press.

Duffy, D.J. (1978) *A Study of Wisconsin Industrial Back Injury Cases*. Madison: University of Wisconsin.

——(1979) Public Attitude Towards Chiropractic and Patient Satisfaction With Chiropractic in the State of Wisconsin. *Journal of Chiropractic* 16(2): 19–24.

Epstein, S.S. (1979) *The Politics of Cancer*. New York: Anchor Press.

FACTS (1980) *Chiropractic Health Care* A National Study of Cost of Education, Service Utilization, Number of Practicing Doctors of Chiropractic, and Other Key Policy Issues, vol. 1. Prepared and Published by the Foundation for the Advancement of Chiropractic Tenets and Science.

Federal Legislation and the Chiropractic Profession (1980) *The Digest of Chiropractic Economics* (January/February): 44, 114.

Firman, G.J. and Goldstein, M.S. (1975) The Future of Chiropractic: A Psychosocial View. *The New England Journal of Medicine* 293(13): 640–41.

Fisk, J.W. (1977) *A Practical Guide to Management of the Painful Neck and Back: Diagnosis, Manipulation, Exercises, Prevention.* Springfield, Ill.: Charles C. Thomas.

Fuchs, V. (1974) *Who Shall Live! Health Economics and Social Choice.* New York: Destiny Books.

Fulder, S. (1980) The Tao of Medicine: Ginseng, Oriental Remedies and the Pharmacology of Harmony. New York: Destiny Books.

Gatterman, M.I. (1981) Contraindications and Complications of Spinal Manipulative Therapy. *ACA Journal of Chiropractic* 15(5): 75ff.

Gerber, A. (1971) *The Gerber Report: The Shocking State of American Medical Care and What Must Be Done About It.* New York: David McKay.

Gibbons, R.W. (1976) The Making of a Chiropractor, 1906 to the Making of a Chiropractic Physician, 1976. *The Digest of Chiropractic Economics* May/June: 99.

——(1979) The Straights Versus the Chiropractors. *International Review of Chiropractic* (October/November): 20ff.

Gold, R.R. (1970) *The Triune of Life.* Davenport, Iowa: ICA Publication.

Gordon, J.S., Hastings A.C., and Fadiman, J. (1981) The Paradigm of Holistic Medicine. In A.C. Hastings, J. Fadiman, and J.S. Gordon *Health for the Whole Person.* New York: Bantam Books.

Haldeman, S. (1976) The Importance of Research in the Principles and Practice of Chiropractic. *JCCA* (October): 7.

——(1980) *Modern Developments in the Principles and Practices of Chiropractic.* New York: Appleton-Century-Crofts.

Hildebrandt, R.W. (1980) Chiropractic Physicians as Members of the Health Care Delivery System: The Case for Increased Utilization. *Journal of Manipulative and Physiological Therapeutics* 3:25.

Hocken, A.G. (1980) Chiropractic in From the Cold? *British Medical Journal* 12 January: 97f.

Hoehler, F., Tobis, J., and Buerger, A. (1981) Spinal Manipulation For Low Back Pain. *JAMA* 245(18): 1835–838.

Horn, J.S. (1969) *Away With All Pests: An English Surgeon in Peoples China 1954–1969.* New York: Monthly Review Press.

Hosek, R., Schram, S., Verman, H., Myers, J., and Williams, S. (1981) Cervical Manipulation. *JAMA* 245(9): 922.

Illich, I. (1976) *Medical Nemesis: The Expropriation of Health.* New York: Pantheon Books.

Inglis, B. (1969) *The Case for Unorthodox Medicine.* New York: Berkley Medallion Books.

——(1979) Breaking the Health Monopoly. *Spectator* 28 July: 14–15.

——(1983) The Alternative Side of the Coin. *The Guardian* 23 March: 11.

Jacobs, M.D. (1980) The Chiropractors' Role in Industry. *Occupational Health and Safety* (October): 67–71.

Jacobs, P. (1980) Ten Chiropractors Named to Medical Review Boards. *Los Angeles Times* 12 January.

Jahn, W.T. (1980) Malpractice in Chiropractic. *The ACA Journal of Chiropractic* (September): 64–7.

Kane, R., Leymaster, C., Olsen, D., Woolley, F., and Fisher, F. (1974) Manipulating the Patient: A Comparison of the Effectiveness of Physician and Chiropractor Care. *The Lancet* 29 June: 1333–336.

Kennedy, E.M. (1972) *In Critical Condition: The Crisis In America's Health Care*. New York: Simon & Schuster.

Kruger, W.J. (1981) Chiropractic Physicians as Members of the Health Care Delivery System. *Journal of Manipulative and Physiological Therapeutics* 4(1): 40.

Kuhn, T.S. (1970) *The Structure of Scientific Revolution*. Chicago: University of Chicago Press.

Kuxhaus, R.L. (1969) *Why Are Medical Doctors Trying to Steal Chiropractic?* Los Angeles: Public Education Publications.

Langone, J. (1982) *Chiropractors: A Consumer's Guide*. Mass: Addison-Wesley.

Levin, L.S., Katz, A.H., and Holst, E. (1976) *Self-Care: Lay Initiatives in Health*. New York: Neale Watson.

Livingston, M.C. (1971) Spinal Manipulation Causing Injury: A Three Year Study. *Clinical Orthopedics* 81: 82–6.

Luce, J.M. (1978) Chiropractic – Its History and Challenge to Medicine. *The Pharos* (April): 12f, 16.

Mackenzie, V. (1978) Fringe Medicine is Beginning to Break Through the Barriers of Medical Scepticism. *The Guardian* 23 June: 9.

Manber, M.M. (1978) Chiropractors: Pushing For A Place On Health Care Team. *Medical World News* 11 December: 58ff.

May, J.J. and Henderson, R.R. (1983) The Business Community Looks at DRG-Based Hospital Reimbursement. *Health Affairs* 2(1): 38–49.

Mazzarelli, J.P. (1982) *Chiropractic: Interprofessional Research*. Torino, Italy: Ed. Izioni, Minerva Medica.

Miller, R.G. (1975) Federal Recognition of Chiropractic: A Double Standard. *Annals of Internal Medicine* 82: 713.

——(1981) History of Chiropractic Accreditation. *ACA Journal of Chiropractic* 18(2): 40.

Mitchell, M. (1980) Maintenance Care: Some Considerations. *ACA Journal of Chiropractic* (April): 53–5.

Modde, R.J. (1979) Malpractice is the Inevitable Result of Chiropractic Philosophy and Training. *Legal Aspects of Medical Practice*: 20–3.

Molthen, D.A. (1968) *The Cause is Chiropractic*. Los Angeles, California: Author Craft Publications.

Moon, D.K. (1981) The Flight From the Subluxation. *ACA Journal of Chiropractic* (November): 22f.

Nofz, M. (1978) Paradigm Indentification and Organizational Structure: An Overview of the Chiropractic Health Care Profession. *The Sociology of Chiropractors and Chiropractic, Sociological Symposium*, Spring, VPI.

O'Bryon, D.S. (1981) Potomac Fever. *ACA Journal of Chiropractic* 18(9): 28–31.

Packo, K. and Shaw, R. (1980) The Future of Chiropractic – Letter to the Editor. *The New England Journal of Medicine* 303(3): 401.

Pelletier, K.R. (1979) *Holistic Medicine: From Stress to Optimum Health.* New York: Delacorte Press.

Potter, G. (1977) A Study of 744 Cases of Neck and Back Pain Treated With Spinal Manipulation. *Journal of Canadian Chiropractic Association* (December): 154–56.

Radovsky, S.S. (1975) Onward With Chiropractic. *The New England Journal of Medicine* 293(13): 662f.

Register of Members [1983]. A pamphlet published by the British Chiropractors' Association, 5 First Avenue, Chelmsford, Essex CM1 1RX.

Research Status of Spinal Manipulative Therapy (1975) Washington, DC: Department of Health Education and Welfare; National Institute of Neurologic and Communicative Disorders and Stroke Monograph 15: National Institutes of Health publication number 76–998.

Relman, A.S. (1979) Chiropractic: Recognized But Unproved. *The New England Journal of Medicine* 301(12): 659–660.

——(1983) The Future of Medical Practice. *Health Affairs* 2(2): 13.

Salmon, J.W. (1982) The Competitive Health Strategy: Fighting For Your Health. *Health and Medicine* 1(2): 21–30.

Salmon, J.W. and Berliner, H. (1982) Self-Care: Boot Straps or Hangman's Noose? *Health and Medicine*, Summer/Fall: 4–11.

Savage, L.J. (1980) A Chiropractic Response. *ACA Journal of Chiropractic*, August: 55–6.

Serafini, A. (1983) The Chiropractic Alternative. *Amtrak Magazine* 3(10): 70–4.

Shearer, A. (1982) Quacks are no Longer Ugly Ducklings. *Guardian*, 7 April: 17.

Sidel, V. and Sidel R. (1983) *A Healthy State.* New York: Pantheon Books.

Silver, G.A. (1980) Chiropractic: Professional Controversy and Public Policy. *American Journal of Public Health* 70(4): 349, 350.

Simons, V. (1980) Chiropractic. In A.C. Hastings, J. Fadiman, and J.S. Gordon *Health For the Whole Person.* New York: Bantam.

Smith, R.L. (1969) *At Your Own Risk: The Case Against Chiropractic.* New York: Pocket Books.

Sobel, D.S. (ed.) (1979) *Ways of Health: Holistic Approaches To Ancient and Contemporary Medicine*. New York: Harcourt Brace Jovanovich.

Starr, P. (1982) *The Social Transformation of American Medicine*. New York: Basic Books.

Suh, C.H., Sharpless, S.K., MacGregor, R.J., Luttges, M.W. (1975) Researching the Fundamentals of Chiropractic. *International Review of Chiropractic* (March): 16–17.

Sullivan, P.H. (1981) Health, Drugs and Chiropractic Values in American Society. *The Digest of Chiropractic Economics* 23(5): 12, 14, 17.

Thomas, L. (1974) *The Lives of a Cell: Notes of a Biology Watcher*. New York: Penguin Books.

Thompson, T.L. (1980) Chiropractic: Recognized But Unproven. *The New England Journal of Medicine* 302(6): 354.

Treaster, J.B. (1978) Chiropractic Comes of Age. *Family Health* 10: 26, 29.

Trever, W. (1972) *In the Public Interest*. Los Angeles, California: Scriptures Unlimited.

Van, J. (1977) Chiropractic: It's Sneered at No Longer. *Chicago Tribune* 9 February.

Verner, J.R., Weiant, C.W., and Watkins, R.J. (1953) *Rational Bacteriology*. Published by authors.

Vogl, A.J. (1974) It's Time to Take Chiropractic Seriously. *Medical Economics* 9 December: 77–81, 84, 85.

Wardwell, W.I. (1976) Orthodox and Unorthodox Practitioners: Changing Relationships and the Future Status of Chiropractors. In R. Wallis and P. Murley (eds) *Marginal Medicine*. New York: The Free Press.

——(1978) Social Factors in the Survival of Chiropractic: A Comparative View. *Sociological Symposium* 22: 6–17.

——(1979) Limited and Marginal Practitioners. In H. Freeman, S. Levine, and L. Reeder (eds) *Handbook of Medical Sociology*, 3rd edn. New Jersey: Prentice-Hall.

——(1980) Sounding Board: The Future of Chiropractic. *The New England Journal of Medicine* 302(12): 688–90.

Webb, E.C. (1977) *Report of the Committee of Inquiry into Chiropractic, Osteopathy, Homeopathy and Naturopathy*. Canberra: Australian Gov. Publ. Service.

Weiskopf, H. (1979) The Good Hands Man. *Sports Illustrated* 51(3): 34–9.

Wiehe, R. (1980) Chiropractic and Third Party Payment. *The Digest of Chiropractic Economics*, Nov/Dec: 62, 65.

Wight, J. (1978) Migraine: A Statistical Analysis of Chiropractic Treatment. *ACA Journal of Chiropractic* 12: 563–67.

Wilk, C.A. (1976) *Chiropractic Speaks Out: A Reply to Medical Propaganda, Bigotry and Ignorance.* Ill.: Wilk Publishing.
——(1980) The New Zealand Report – A Summary. *The Digest of Chiropractic Economics* March/April: 47–8, 50–1.
Williams, A.G. (1980) The Future of Chiropractic: Letter to the Editor. *The New England Journal of Medicine* 303(7): 400.
Yesalis, C., Wallace, R., Fisher, W., and Tokheim, R. (1980) Does Chiropractic Utilization Substitute for Less Available Medical Services? *American Journal of Public Health* 70: 415–17.

Four

Traditional Chinese medicine: a holistic system

Effie Poy Yew Chow

Introduction

This chapter attempts to highlight the development of traditional Chinese medicine, its philosophical and theoretical tenets, its status and some policy implications in the People's Republic of China, the UK, and the US. This is intended as a basic introduction to a unique system which requires arduous, specialized training of its practitioners.

Because of the particular focus on acupuncture, and to some extent, herbology, in the US and China, the information presented here emphasizes these branches of Chinese medicine. However, two things must be understood in connection with the fact that Chinese medicine is not yet well known in the west. First, acupuncture and herbology are but two branches in a very large system. Second, the response in the US and the western hemisphere to the science of acupuncture should be taken as representative of response in the west to traditional Chinese medicine *as a whole*.

Although western science is today making some attempts at analysis of these theories, the differences in language and philosophical concepts have posed a formidable barrier for understanding the enormous value of traditional Chinese medicine. In this connection, it should be pointed out that terminologies and spellings in this chapter vary in different texts. For example Chi is interchangeably written as Ch'i, Chh'i, or Qi; the Five Phases are often called the Five Elements. But they refer none the less to the same basic phenomenology, regardless of these variations.

Traditional Chinese medicine is first and foremost a holistic system in which health is understood as the cooperative functioning parts within a context. History and principles in Chinese medicine are inseparable. The fundamental concepts are embedded in Confucianism and Taoism which by 600 BC stood as two fully evolved philosophies. The Taoist branch came to have enormous influence on the traditional art of healing. Taoism was a conception of the universe as a cosmogony of endlessly moving components, all of which were aspects of the same unity, the same reality.

> There are the three terms: "complete," "all-embracing," "the whole." These names are different, but the reality sought in them is the same: referring to the One Thing.
> (*Chuang Tzu*: Chapter 22)

The highest code of conduct was to act spontaneously in accordance with the Tao, or one's own nature, for they were the same. The ancients were said to have followed the guidance of the sages who educated them in, among other things, disease prevention. It was said "The ancient sages did not treat those who were already ill; they instructed those who were not ill" (Veith 1970: 53).

In observing the interplay of the polarities in nature, the sages intuited Yin and Yang, the primordial pair of opposites. This is the basic principle which guides and informs the movements of the Tao and constitutes, as well, the seminal principle of Chinese medical theory. These opposites were perceived in a dynamic interplay in which they cease to be opposites and become each other. There is always Yin in Yang and Yang in Yin, a fundamental unity expressed in the *Chuang Tzu* as:

> The "This" is also "that." The "that" is also "This." . . .

That the "that" and the "this" cease to be opposites is the very essence of Tao. Only this essence, an axis as it were, is the center of the circle corresponding to the endless Changes. (Fung Yu-lan 1964:112)

The first mention of Yin–Yang was in the first millennium BC in the *I Ching* (The Book of Changes). As a philosophical work, the *I Ching* had a profound influence on Chinese medical thought in so far as it posited ideas of opposition, transmutation, and patterns in motion. In the *I Ching*, Yin was delineated as negative, dark, cold, feminine and Yang meant positive, light, warm, masculine. Later additional important meanings were contractive and downward flowing (Yin) and expansive and flowing upward and outward (Yang). All things in the universe could be categorized as Yin or Yang. These pair of opposites carried no connotation of bad or good any more than a negatively or positively charged ion is bad or good. Yin and Yang was in actuality, an elegant "two-pole model" (Wei 1979a: 73) developed by the ancients in order to construct a body of theory which would be consistent.

Chinese medical thinking was predicated on two other major principles in addition to Yin–Yang, namely, Chi or vital energy, and the Five Phases doctrine. Chi meant originally "air," "ether," or "breath." By the first century AD, it had taken on the meaning of what Stephan Palos calls the "original material substance" which creates the universe and everything in it. In the human body, it was perceived as the supreme nourishing and protective principle. It circulated through the meridians, or channels, and activated the energy in the circulatory system. The respiratory exercises, Chi Kung, and the martial art, Tai Chi Chuan were to stimulate the flow of Chi in the channels.

Fritjof Capra (1975: 199–200) detects a "striking resemblance" between the traditional notion of Chi as the primal creative energy as a subtle form of matter and the quantum field in modern physics. In a similar vein, S. Mahdihassan makes the following comparison from physics:

It is consistent to attribute the source of all creation to *Chhi* for, being matter-plus-energy, every form of matter, like water, plant and man, can be traced to it, as can every form of energy such as heat and light. But with all that we cannot conceive what *Chhi* actually is. Now in physics there is the corpuscular theory of light, implying that light is matter-plus-energy. *Chhi* then would be corpuscular creative energy, containing far more energy than matter.

(Mahdihassan 1982: 273)

Chi then was regarded as an amalgam of "both matter and energy", that is, it has the attributes of both (Shanghai College of Traditional Medicine 1981: 2). Chi, in fact, meant nothing less than Cosmic Soul or Consciousness.

The Five Phases, wood, fire, earth, metal, and water (sometimes called the Five Elements) were actually sub-classifications of Yin and Yang. They were the microcosmic or material components of this principle and, like Yin–Yang, represented a cycle of creation and subjugation, or production (Yang) and conquest (Yin), in a continuum of exchange of states of being. Their importance lay not in the elements, as such, but in the way they changed and interacted with the rest of the system. Each of the elements in this doctrine connects to any of the other four (Wei 1979b: 79). Thus as metal creates water (liquefies), and water creates wood, so conversely, wood destroys earth (absorbs nutrients), earth destroys water (absorbs or dams it), water destroys fire, fire destroys metal, and metal destroys wood (an axe fells trees).

The Five Phases doctrine was used historically to classify any category of things or qualities, such as color, sound, taste, emotions, weather, the planets, animals, etc. As well, the Five Phases were applied to the internal organs, suggesting complex functional interrelationships between all organs which are classified as Yin and Yang organs. The integral position of the Five Phases in the Chinese medical system may be illustrated by the following: since each of the Yin or Yang organs are associated with wood, fire, earth, metal, or water, this means that, for example, in acupuncture therapy, two organs are usually treated; that is, not only the affected organ is treated, but also the one that is *next in sequence* in the Five Phases energy cycle (Palos 1972: 47–8).

Systemic relationships such as these were recorded over a period of three thousand years in Chinese medical texts. In the sense that there exists this exhaustive clinical record which has documented patterns of correlations and processes in the human body, some modern scientists believe that the Five

Phases has enormous potential in explaining organic functions especially in conjunction with modern medical research.

Some major ancient medical texts

The ancient medical literature was marked by two distinguishing features. First, the Chinese were preoccupied with the careful observation of nature and the cosmos. Ko Hung (281–340 BC), one of the great Han Dynasty alchemists, retired to the mountains after a brilliant military career there to observe nature, or the Tao. A renowned physician, he produced treatises in pathology, internal medicine, and medication.

In addition to observation, the Chinese had a scientific approach with regard to the complementary procedural steps of analysis, deduction, and interpretation. Centuries before Christ (Chou Dynasty 1066–221 BC), Chinese medicine was already highly developed and organized. The state "distinguished four kinds of doctors: namely, physicians, surgeons, dietitians and veterinary surgeons. . . . Careful clinical records were kept, and such facts as vital statistics and cause of death were also recorded" (Kao 1979: 7). Doctors belonged to the civil branch of government and their work was evaluated annually.

The Great Herbal, *Pen Tsao*, which evolved in 3000 BC, listed 365 herbs including their properties. It was probably compiled by several authors, but is attributed to Shen Nung, the Father of Chinese Medicine.

The treatment methods of Pien Chiao (500 BC) typified the ancient holistic practice, namely: diagnosis by means of auscultation and osphresiology, amnesis, and pulse diagnosis (sphygmology); and treatment methods which included acupuncture, moxibustion, aqueous or alcoholic decoctions of drugs, massage, gymnastics, medical plasters, and surgery (the latter atypical in later centuries) (Kao 1979: 11).

The undisputed classic of traditional medicine is the *Huang Ti Nei Ching: The Yellow Emperor's Classic of Internal Medicine*. It's estimated to have been compiled throughout the first millennium BC and recorded in the first century. Its principles and therapies had evolved in earlier millennia, however, reputedly beginning with the reign of the Yellow Emperor

(2697 BC). This classic is a compendium of physiological and experiential knowledge which expounds on the organs and their functions and interrelationships in accordance with their respective Yin–Yang natures and the Five Phases and which discourses on diagnostics, acupuncture, dietetics, and breathing.

By the beginning of the Han Dynasty (200 BC), the Chinese had acquired a formidable medical experience. They practiced sophisticated surgery (laparotomies, grafting of organs, intestinal resections, etc.) and anesthesiology (Huard and Wong 1968: 19), although in later centuries the Confucian belief of the sacredness of the human body prevented surgery as well as anatomical research. In China, "the circulation of blood and ch'i was standard doctrine in the second century" (Lu and Needham 1980: 29). During the same period the surgeon Ha T'o developed anatomical charts, practiced pharmacology, used hydrotherapy, and invented the physical exercise therapy Wu-Chin-Hi, the Game of the Five Animals (tiger, stag, bear, monkey, and crane). In this therapy, "the *Niao-Hi* (the bird game) facilitates breathing. The arms are spread out as the bird raises its wings. The monkey game (*Yuan-Hi*) teaches the art of climbing, and so forth" (Huard and Wong 1968: 19). The ancient theory of pulse diagnosis was also synthesized during this early period by the physician Wan Shu Ho.

By the close of the Han period, the Chinese had a clear idea of preventive medicine and first aid, knew pathology and dietetics, had devised a respiratory therapy, and had formulated "a mental technique (e.g. Taoist philosophy) which radiated through Eurasia" (Huard and Wong 1968: 35). By 600–700 AD, there had appeared the first materia medica and works on ophthalmology, obstetrics, acupuncture, dental treatment, and orthopedics. There was a national ministry of health and a public health system.

The Tang Sung period (618–907 AD) saw the invention of printing, the flourishing of Buddhism, and the creation of the life-sized bronzes, or acupuncture mannequins, of Wang Wei.

In the sixteenth century, the *Great Herbal* or *Materia-Medica* was written by Li Shih-chen, which Needham has compared with the accomplishments of Newton. A monumental work on infectious diseases was published in 1642. The author, Wu You-Ke was aware of an external causal agent, i.e. "bacteria" (Kao 1979: 22).

After 1822, internal political factors precipitated the adoption of western medicine and the discontinuance of traditional methods. They were revived in 1949 when Chairman Mao directed the amalgamation of the two streams. This signaled a remarkable period of integration of the traditional and western schools into "one universal physical system." More will be said about this at a later point.

Diagnosis and treatment

It will be helpful here to bring the philosophical concept of Yin–Yang into more specific focus as a principle in the Chinese art of healing and to define the Ching–Lo doctrine or system of meridians.

The basic role of Yin–Yang in human health is simply that when their harmony is disrupted there is illness, and when they are in good balance, there is health. One example of the law of Yin–Yang balance in physical health is the pH balance of body fluids as being either more acidic (Yang) or more alkaline (Yin) (Wei 1979b: 75). In terms of the displacement of body energy, Yang means hyperactivity and Yin hypoactivity. The traditional therapies are used to disperse *or* tonify in order to correct such imbalances.

Globally speaking, the body surface is Yang, the inside Yin, and the front (chest and abdomen) is Yin, the back Yang. Internal organs are also Yin or Yang. The Yin, or "solid" organs, are the liver, heart, spleen, lungs, and kidneys. The Yang, or "hollow" organs are the gall-bladder, small intestine, stomach, large intestine, and bladder. And there are many other finer determinants of Yin and Yang.

The central structural system of traditional Chinese medicine is a "network model" (Wei 1979b: 73) of twelve major channels or meridians and their collaterals, or branches, in which the vital energy (Chi) circulates. Well-defined points on the body surface connect with the internal viscera and parts of the body. The points affect particular organs such that a Yin meridian emanates from a Yin organ and Yang meridian from a Yang organ. Each of the Yin meridians is connected with a Yang channel at the hand or foot. There are, in addition, eight extra meridians, each having its own set of points. The channels

(Chings) are longitudinal and conjunct with neighboring channels through short, horizontal collaterals or branches (Lo).

Diagnosis

The overriding theme of the ancient life style was the harmony of the human microcosm with macrocosmic laws. One should not eat or sleep too much or too little, nor consume an excess of Yin or Yang foods. To expose oneself to extreme temperatures would be "rebellion" against the principle of harmonious interaction with the atmosphere of the five seasons. The power of acting in accordance with the Right Way was inestimable: "Even a heavy storm, afflictions or poison, cannot injure those people who live in accord with the natural order" (Veith 1970: 107).

The first level of cure in earliest times was spiritual redirection. Diagnostic methods were said to have evolved with the development of a more complex civilization and its human demands. However, diagnosis remained functionally preventive in nature, that is, it was performed on a regular basis to detect whether the balance of Yin–Yang forces was harmonious, and to discern their precise effect on the course of the Chi. Consequently, the Chinese physician himself became a refined instrument in the combined diagnostic/prognostic procedure.

Diagnosis involves four procedures: looking, listening, questioning, and feeling the pulse (sphygmology). Chinese medicine advocates the use of all four procedures together, one by itself being inadequate. Looking and listening are lucid (ming); sphygmology is intelligent (shen); and questioning workmanlike (chung). To use only one diagnostic method is chung, to use two is shen, to use all, both shen and ming (Huard and Wong 1968: 193–94). The *Nei Ching* dwells on the need of accuracy in the diagnostic procedures: diagnosis must eliminate all "doubt or confusion" so that "no mistakes or neglect occur" (Veith 1970: 57). Ideally, the diagnosis should be performed in early morning (Yin and rising Yang) when physician and patient are uncontaminated by the intake of substances or by worldly distractions.

The physician first inspects the body orifices and the tongue for their color, tone, texture, odor, and temperature. The soles of the feet and the palms of the hands, nails, and hair are observed for any telling characteristics such as perspiration, texture, color, and topography. There are no less than one hundred different conditions of the tongue including color (purplish, yellowish, blackish, etc.), topography, or specific location (back, front, tip, sides, underside, etc.). Similarly, urine and feces are analyzed for color, odor, volume, and frequency or retention. In listening, the physician carefully observes the sound of the breathing, sighing, or coughing since the manner of inhalation and exhalation is associated with particular organs and bodily functions.

In questioning the patient, the physician searches for details of habit, style of life, and specific mediating circumstances. Dreams as well reveal internal physiological conditions, for example, "Fullness of the lungs produces dreams of sorrow and weeping."

Taking the pulse is an exacting process which is thought of as providing the deepest, most subtle information. Traditionally, there are eighteen pulses. In twelve of these, each is associated with one of the twelve organ systems or a physiologic area. Chinese physicians take pulses of the neck and leg arteries as well as the wrists, but the radial artery of the forearms is the seat of a refined, complex diagnostic system. The eighteen pulses are located nine on each radial pulse area, each with a specific name, and capable of recording the pathology of a physiologic location. Measured against one inhalation and exhalation of his own breath, the physician takes four pulse beats as the norm. He knows the normal sounds of the pulses as well as their pathological aberrations *or* seasonal fluctuations. The four basic patterns, which vary in accordance with their corresponding organs and the person's health, can possess twenty-eight different qualities. The lung pulse should sound soft as "hair or feathers blowing in the wind," but the heart pulse should have the "ringing sound of a sickle," first strong and clear and then "trailing off" (Wallnöfer and von Rottauscher 1972: 100). If the pulse of heart or lung beats "vigorously and long and the strokes are markedly prolonged," the patient is ill. If pulse beats associated with the various organs coincide in certain combination, this indicates a *specific* ailment. Gradations of imbalances are often extremely fine and identified by terms such as choking, tender, limping, wavering, tangled as weed.

Some western physicians are now beginning to recognize the efficacy of sphygmology as a diagnostic/prognostic tool. Chinese physicians, however, continue to advocate its use more for prevention than for crisis intervention.

Traditional treatment methodologies

Limitations of space prohibit detailed discussion of traditional treatment methodologies, but it is possible to outline the major therapies and indicate something of their current usage. All have evolved from earliest times and all are based on the principles of Yin–Yang, the Five Phases, and the flow of vital energy, Chi. The power and accuracy of these theories are now being increasingly validated in the light of new research.

Acupuncture   It is important to remember that acupuncture is but one branch among several therapies. It is perhaps the most direct of the manipulative therapies in that the network of meridians which connect with deeper internal organs and other body parts are precisely outlined and accessible. Acupuncture, acupressure, and moxibustion, are used to redirect and normalize the flow of Chi. Acupuncture is the insertion of fine needles into surface points. Today some 722 points are well known, the commonly used number is between forty and fifty. However, new points are continually being rediscovered so that there is an ongoing re-evaluation.

The needle is manipulated to disperse or reactivate the Chi. Tonifying or dispersing depending on the method of insertion – quick, intermittent, rotated, or insertion which is synchronized with breathing are some major examples.

Professor Xi Yong-jiang, Chief of the Acupuncture Department of the Shanghai College of Traditional Chinese Medicine reports that acupuncture therapy is used for acute conditions, including the following: abdominal pain, abdominal disease, urinary tract infection, conjunctivitis, hepatitis, acute nephritis, viral diarrhoea, gastro-intestinal enteritis, malaria, asthma, biliary pain of duct, renal kidney pain, and acute urinary tract blockage.

There are a number of western theories which attempt to account for the successes of acupuncture therapy. In neurophysiological terms, the needles are thought to stimulate the receptors at various depths which then send impulses to the brain via the spinal cord. Acupuncture therapy strengthens the patient's resistance, perhaps by increasing antibody production, but not by directly attacking the invading foreign element, not in other words, by the " 'antiseptic' attack" characteristic of western medicine (Lu and Needham 1980: 607). Ling Wei, in an important article on recent scientific advance in acupuncture (Kao 1979: 66), likewise proposes that acupuncture somehow "raises the body defense-mechanism" and puts it "back in order". For this reason he believes it holds tremendous promise for immunology.

Nakatani's discovery (Kyoto University 1950) that certain points on the meridians when measured electrically for skin resistance have lower resistance when the person is in an unhealthy state established a linkage between the meridians and the autonomic nervous system. This discovery supports the Ching-Lo doctrine as it is described in the *Huang-Ti Nei Ching* (Wei 1979a: 52). Rheinhold Voll in Germany has developed a similar technique (using electro-acupuncture) for diagnosis and therapy.

Acupuncture analgesia has generated enormous interest in China and the west. Chang Hsiang-Tung and his group (Shanghai Psychological Institute) have pioneered in this area of neurophysiology since the mid 1960s and have definitely demonstrated the physical manifestation of pain, within a certain frequency spectrum, in the thalamus of the brain as well as the inhibitory effects of acupuncture on these "pain discharge waves" (Wei 1979a: 55).

Research on the relationship of acupuncture and pain has centered around the theory of "gating" – the effort to find the points of intersection of the pain signal and acupuncture stimulation points. The notion of a "gate control" theory was first proposed in 1965 by Melzack and Wall. Recent research in Shanghai indicates that one of the central "control" locations is in the medulla.

A major breakthrough in studies of an "opiate" in the brain released by acupuncture was the discovery, in the mid 1970s, that enkephalin-endorphin levels in the cerebrospinal fluid *increased* as pain response *decreased* (Lu and Needham 1980: 260–61). The relationship with analgesia by means of acupuncture is that the nerve stimulation resulting from acupuncture may "trigger" the release of endorphins (pain-inhibiting chemicals) from the pituitary gland. Considerable research is in progress on pain threshold variations induced by acupuncture in two related areas of study: (1) studies of a natural analgesic substance produced in the brain by acupuncture, and (2) comparative studies of artificially introduced analgesic chemicals such as morphine and a "morphine-like factor" produced in the brain by acupuncture (Lu and Needham 1980: 256).

For several decades the Chinese have researched the effects of acupuncture on blood. Their findings reveal that acupuncture stimulation affects certain centers which regulate blood content activity (phagocytic activity and fibrinolytic activity). Still other research in China reveals that acupuncture can reduce blood pressure (Wei 1979a: 62). Recently, Ionescu-Tirgoriste and Mincu have had favorable response in the treatment of diabetes.

Auriculotherapy has been an important application of acupuncture theory and treatment since it was developed by Nogier in 1950. Nogier mapped the external ear as a projection of the various internal organs and developed complementary diagnostic and therapeutic techniques which include acupuncture. The use of acupuncture points in the ear has been markedly successful in treating drug addiction, obesity, and pain in the spinal column and limbs (Wei 1979a: 64).

Some scientists see potential applications for acupuncture in new areas, for example, circadian rhythms. The "biological clock" or natural rhythmic patterns peculiar to the individual internal organs are believed to be amenable to regulation through acupuncture (Wei 1979a: 66).

In China, acupuncture has been used in over a million painless surgical procedures, including pulmonary lobectomies, heart surgery, Caesarian sections, and various abdominal operations (Kao 1979: 35). Today it is the method of choice in 15 to 30 per cent of all surgical cases (Lu and Needham 1980: 22). Beyond this, it continues to be a major treatment modality in the fusion of Chinese traditional and western scientific medicine.

Acupressure Acupressure treatment uses the same points as in acupuncture except that pressure is applied in this case with the fingertips. The method has long been used in China and

Japan (Shiatsu) and is now becoming popular in the United States. Kurland (1977) has reported extraordinary results with the use of acupressure for pain. The obvious advantages of this therapy are that it is safe, painless, without side effects, effective in a wide variety of illness, and easy to learn. Acupressure and Shiatsu techniques are now available in a growing library of published materials in the US, Namikoshi's and deLangre's work among them.

Moxibustion Acupuncture and moxibustion are complementary techniques and are often applied at the same time. Moxibustion is forbidden at certain points, just as acupuncture is forbidden at certain other points.

Moxibustion evolved in earliest times in northern China, a cold, mountainous region where the vasodilative effects on the skin by heating were a logical development. It is thought to have preceded the use of surgical needles. The term *moxa* derives from the Japanese name of the plant *Artemesia vulgaris* of the chrysanthemum family. The plant must be grown nine years to achieve the correct maturity. Mugwort is also a commonly used leaf.

In modern moxibustion treatment, burning moxa sticks made of the rolled leaves are held over the energy points in dosages which vary anywhere from 3 to 20 minutes. This action produces heat which penetrates, deeply affecting the flow of Chi. A dispersive or tonifying effect may be achieved by different movements of the moxa stick. In the older traditional form of moxibustion treatment, moxa cones are placed on the energy point and lit from the top so that a pleasant warmth is created in the vacuum.

Remedial massage The techniques of remedial massage, *An-Mo* and *Tui-na*, are described in medical texts of the Han period. Later (in the Tang Dynasty) massage was taught in special institutes. *An-Mo* tonifies by "pressing and rubbing" while *Tui-Na* soothes and sedates by "thrusting and rolling" hand motions. Both systems employ a complex system of hand movements (the eight Kua) on specific body areas in order to produce a desired effect on corresponding organs and organ functions. In China, the simpler hand movements are common practice among family members. The movements are used in reducing fever, to sedate, to alleviate nausea and diarrhoea, to relieve emotional trauma, and to treat bronchitis and influenza (Palos).

Cupping   Cupping is used in the treatment of arthritis, bronchitis, and sprains, among other ailments. Heated jars are applied to body points in order to disperse congestion. The technique involves creating a vacuum in the jar by first warming and then attaching it by suction over the selected point(s) for ten to fifteen minutes. In treating bronchitis, medicinal herbs can be placed in the cup along with the heating substance. In lung congestion, the jar is attached to the point(s) on the chest or back nearest the congestion.

Respiratory exercise   The centrality of the breath in physical therapy appeared in inscribed form on jade stones dated the sixth century BC which were excavated in archaeological finds:

> In breathing we must proceed as follow. One holds the breath and it is collected together. If it is collected, it expands. When it expands it goes down. When it goes down, it becomes quiet. When it becomes quiet, it will solidify. When it becomes solidified, it will begin to sprout. After it has sprouted, it will grow. As it grows, it will be pulled back again to the upper region. When it has been pulled back, it will reach the crown of the head. Above, it will press against the crown of the head. Below, it will press downwards. Whoever follows this will live; whoever acts contrary to it will die.

Historically, in every early form of physical exercise, breathing and mental training were incorporated in physical culture – whose ultimate purpose, like the other therapies, was to regulate the circulation of the breath and blood (Chi). Before performing the actual gymnastics of the Five Animals exercises, for example, a week had to be spent concentrating on breathing (Chi Kung) to free the mind of all "wandering thoughts." Chi Kung was also used in classical forms of Tai Chi and boxing. Professional boxers used deep breathing and breath conduction (taking the breath below the navel) as mechanisms to stop heartbeats and take blows without pain.

The state of being that occurs when respiratory exercise is

done correctly cannot be objectively defined. It must be sub-jectively experienced. Three basic principles are observed in the performance of the exercises: relaxation and repose (Sung Chung Wei Chu); association of breathing with attention (I-chi Hi); and the interaction of movement and rest (Lien-yang Hsiang-chien). In China, these exercises are taught by skilled therapists in institutional settings.

Physical exercise   Tai Chi and other practices of Chinese physical culture constitute the art of maintaining internal and external balance while in movement. Gymnastics was named after the Tai Chi symbol, the "Diagram of the Supreme Ulti-mate," which graphically represents the continuous cyclic movement of Yin and Yang, the dots in the symbol signifying the seed of the one in the other. Thus in Tai Chi gymnastics, the exercises are done in a circular fashion. The limbs move like the "four wheels of a wagon" with the trunk and hips as the axles in the continuous flowing motions of a river (Huard and Wong 1968: 224).

Because the goal of physical exercise is to produce and circu-late vital energy, it has the overall name Chi Kung, or "prepara-tion of Chi." All exercise, regardless of form, involves the use of the inner breath (Nei-Chung) and outer muscle strengthening (Chian-Chuang-Kung). Essentially, there must be a synthesis of inner and outer work: deep, quiet breathing combined with effortlessness; equilibrium, or a prepared center of gravity; flowing movement like "cattle chewing cud"; continuous momentum; and alternate movements of upper and lower (i.e. arms and legs) are basic principles (Palos 1972: 168–69). Of all the martial arts, Tai Chi is the most accomplished.

> In terms of the focus of the inner eye. EEG studies have shown that merely mentally rehearsing the movements of Tai Chi Chuan, not only increased the duration of the alpha rhythm, but produced gradually increasing theta waves – believed to be evidence of decreased excitability in the cere-bral cortex.   (Zhuo 1982: 286)

The number of movements varies depending on the school. The modified Chin School, as taught by Kuo Lien Lee, consists of 64 movements; the Yang Tai Chi has over 200 movements: a third school has only 38. It has been noted that there are over 100 styles.

Herb medicine Pharmacological records begin with the oracle bones of pre-Christian millennia (thirteenth/fourteenth centuries). In the seventh century, the *Pharmacopoeia* of Shen Nung listed 844 items.

Some commonly used Chinese herbs and their properties follow;

Acontium uncinatium, Tsao Wu Tou, (or clambering monkshood) contains a highly toxic substance which, used appropriately, reduces fever and acts as a local pain-reliever when applied superficially.

Panax ginseng, Gen Shen, alone or in combination, has literally hundreds of applications: for depression, to stimulate circulation, for insomnia, stiffness in the joints, sexual excess, nausea, menstrual disorders, vascular disorders, rheumatism.

Angelica polymorpha, Tang Kuei, is highly regarded as a blood cleanser and for menstrual disorders and hemorrhoids, among other ailments. It is the female equivalent of ginseng.

Orange peel is used in sedative prescriptions and the willow for rheumatism.

There are complex laws governing the preparation and administering of herbs. In ancient times, as today, pharmacology required a long apprenticeship and internship. In addition to knowledge of the body's Yin–Yang balance, the therapist must have knowledge of Chi and Ching-Lo for purposes of diagnosis and treatment. Herbal prescriptions are usually selected for their action upon particular meridians and might be used in conjunction with moxa or acupuncture. There is also a special connection between herbs and Five Phases theory, specifically with regard to the five kinds of taste: sour, bitter, sweet, sharp, salty and their relationships with particular internal organs.

Herbology requires, in addition, the subtlest understanding of how to use and combine ambivalent and polyvalent herbs; e.g. *Atractylis* and licorice combine harmoniously so as to purge without injury (Huard and Wong 1968: 197). Certain prescriptions have to be both tonic and dispersive; the toxic component can become effective only after a balancing ingredient has dispersed a potentially perverse effect. Toxins can also be neutralized by combining them with an antidote.

Chinese herbs in traditional medicine are arranged in a hierarchy of "ruler," "minister," "deputy," and "delegate," or "servant," that is in a hierarchy of a master and associate drugs. Many conductors, for example, promote therapeutic results by *facilitating* the master remedy. The general strategy was to promote beneficial results and inhibit, or neutralize undesirable effects.

A new pharmacology is presently being developed in China. Herbs are seen everywhere in the rural communes and in the gardens of urban medical schools (Kao 1979: 34). A large group of plants is under study, including antimalarial drugs, a uterine haemostatic, analgesics, antibiotics, and a substitution for insulin from *Panax ginseng*. The latter is widely used as a cardiac tonic in China (Li 1975: 216). Anti-toxic and anti-inflammatory herb medicine is being used for acute abdominal conditions along with acupuncture (Kao 1979: 33). Bronchitis is treated almost exclusively with herbs (about 150 varieties).

Biomedical scientists in China have collected and identified more than 2,000 herbs during the last quarter century. These are being analyzed both as single agents and in compound prescriptions. Ephedrine is one example of a new isolate (Li 1975: 215); another is anisodamine which is being used successfully in microcirculatory disturbances in the incipient stages of acute infections such as septic shock and in fulminant bacterial epidemic meningitis (Li 1975: 216).

Traditional Chinese medicine in modern China

A vast new literature of Chinese contemporary medicine has developed in China. Much of this involves the investigation of arcane Chinese medical theory. This, in turn, is helping produce a truly ecumenical east/west medical science. Medical personnel of both western and traditional medical schools in China not only continue their medical studies in the institutions of the opposite tradition, but there is also a steadily growing trend of combining the Chinese and western traditions in the closest proximity such that the two types of physicians have joint consultations and clinical examinations (Lu and Needham 1980: 3).

Interestingly, the Chinese are emphasizing the holistic

nature of traditional Chinese medicine through their extensive research in ancient texts. Traditional theories of physiology, etiology, and pathology along with their methodological principles and practices are seen as constituting "a unified whole with methodology as the pivot" (Li 1975: 216). The traditional methodologies or therapeutic principles are found to reveal not only the "action" of an application – for example, of a prescription – but also to illuminate the nature of the disease and the direction of its diagnosis and treatment.

Traditional Chinese medicine in the United Kingdom

Although there has been earlier identified interest in the UK, a major wave of interest in acupuncture began in the late eighteenth century and the first half of the nineteenth century. Among the first practitioners were Doctors Jukes and Coley. While the first great protagonist was J.M. Churchill who published two books on it, his successes were mostly with what he called "local diseases of the muscular and fibrous structures of the body" (Lu and Needham 1980: 297) This interest waned in the last half of the nineteenth century until the next period of major interest was observed in the mid-twentieth century, in the 1950s and 1960s.

The only school in the early 1960s was the College of Chinese Acupuncture of the United Kingdom in Oxford under Jack Worsley. Many people who did not study at this school went to Taiwan and studied under Wu Wei Ping (Daniels 1984 interview). In the late 1960s a branch of this College became the British College of Acupuncture in London under Dr Van Buren. In 1978 the original College was renamed The College of Traditional Acupuncture. Subsequently a branch of this college was instituted as the first Acupuncture clinic and school in Columbia, Maryland in the US.

Acupuncture training in England was provided under the auspices of the trade schools and no special licensing was required. Currently this remains the same, but there are attempts to place acupuncture training under the Ministry of Education. The practice of acupuncture has been under the jurisdiction of the Board of Trade. However, in response to the US controversial status on acupuncture in the 1970s, a sense of caution also arose in the UK. Attempts are being made to restrict acupuncture as a practice of medicine with licensing requirements and under the surveillance of the British Medical Association.

These actions are going through political processes. The outcome is not apparent at this point, but organizations interested in preserving the independence and quality of acupuncture are springing up. Two better known ones are the Traditional Acupuncture Society in Marwood, Barnstaple and the British Acupuncture Association in London.

Traditional Chinese medicine in the United States

The status of traditional Chinese medicine in the US is plagued with problems stemming primarily from the failure to distinguish Chinese and western medicine as different systems. There are consequently no uniform standards under which to practice and teach the Chinese healing arts. This situation is beginning to be somewhat ameliorated by the passage of legislation in approximately a dozen states, accomplished in large part by acupuncture organizations and clienteles.

The American Association of Acupuncture and Oriental Medicine (AAAOM) is a newly created umbrella organization to coordinate research and legislative efforts of acupuncture organizations nationwide. The North American Acupuncture Association (NAAA) which publishes the newsletter *The American Acupuncturist* in conjunction with the AAAOM, serves as a communication network and offers insurance benefits. The AAAOM has worked assiduously for open communication among acupuncture organizations such as The Tri-State Institute of Traditional Medicine, Midwest Center for the Study of Oriental Medicine, The Traditional Acupuncture Institute, the New England School of Acupuncture, The California Acupuncture College, The San Francisco College of Acupuncture, Samra University, and other schools.

In 1982, in a landmark event, thirteen fully established US residential programs offering a minimum of a two-year entry level competency program in traditional acupuncture formed the National Council of Acupuncture Schools and Colleges

(NCASC). Functioning autonomously, an NCASC commission is currently accepting applications for accreditation from two-year residential programs. Further, the NCASC has set up a Certification Task Force to pursue the important work of establishing a National Board of Examination in acupuncture. Some states foresee the possibility of purchasing such an exam so as to license independent practitioners when lobbying efforts in the state lead to passage of bills mandating such examinations (*The American Acupuncturist* March 1983 2(1): 1). To a large extent, the matter of who can practice acupuncture rests with boards of medical examiners in each state since the state boards play an authoritative role regarding the legal status of acupuncture.

State requirements for practicing acupuncture vary extremely. The majority of the states (about forty) restrict practice solely to physicians and doctors of osteopathic medicine. In some cases, their assistants – trained acupuncturists – are permitted to practice under physician supervision. California, Florida, Hawaii, Montana, Nevada, New Jersey, and New York have state board requirements which allow trained and properly educated acupuncturists to practice independently. However, educational requirements, even among this group, vary widely. Montana, for instance, requires a total of 105 hours in anatomy, biochemistry, microbiology or bacteriology, pharmacology, physiology, chemistry, and materia medica, but requires no training in traditional Chinese medicine. Nevada, on the other hand, requires three years of acupuncture training (1,400 hours or more) plus three years of practice, and requires that both physicians and nonphysicians pass an examination in acupuncture and traditional Chinese medicine.

Texas and Oklahoma allow independent practice of acupuncture, but require no formal evidence whatever of training or education. In Utah, acupuncture practice is considered illegal. However, as of the spring of 1983, Utah appears to be "on the brink" of passage of acupuncture legislation perhaps utilizing the NCASC acupuncture exam as the state exam. This would be a major breakthrough in standardizations procedure in the US (*The American Acupuncturist* March 1983 2(1): 1).

Of the fifty states, roughly fourteen require varying amounts of special education and training for physicians (includes DOs) and/or independent practitioners: California, Florida, Georgia,

Hawaii, Louisiana, Maryland, Montana, Nevada, New York, New Jersey, Oregon, Virginia, and Washington (Rhode Island and Utah have pending legislation). The rest of the states, according to a 1981 survey conducted by the Traditional Acupuncture Foundation in Columbia, Maryland, do not mention any requirement for educational preparation for the practice of acupuncture.

As long as a decade ago, Nevada was the pacesetter in both legislation and state board requirements. It was the first state to establish a special state Board of Chinese Medicine in recognition of acupuncture and its complementary modalities as a different treatment system with its own set of definitions, terminologies, and delivery system. It was also the first to require both physicians and nonphysicians to pass an examination in acupuncture and traditional medicine. Of major importance, in addition, is that Nevada's Chinese Medicine Act is not limited to the practice of acupuncture. Since the law encompasses broad aspects of Chinese medicine, licenses can be granted to practitioners of traditional Chinese medicine, herbal medicine, acupuncture, or, to acupuncture assistants after completion of examinations in the appropriate subject. Further, the law states that the board may waive examination and grant a certificate of Doctor of Traditional Chinese Medicine to any applicant who has a certificate from either the Republic of China, Korea, Japan, or the People's Republic of China, if the applicant has been qualified to practice Chinese medicine for at least ten years immediately prior to the effective date of the act.

Clearly, the current status of legislation in many states creates considerable turmoil for both acupuncturists and consumers. The non-western medical doctor acupuncturist, particularly, is confronted with a complex of legal, medical, and professional dilemmas, and the consumers themselves are often forced to seek acupuncture treatment from either illegal or inexperienced practitioners. In most cases acupuncture treatment is not reimbursed by third party payment, private insurance, or public-supported benefits. In addition, recipients of acupuncture training, including medical doctors, are too often being provided with inadequate and limited courses. Many, unfortunately, are led to believe that the brief training they receive qualifies them as acupuncturists. In the majority of states, acupuncturists who practice privately are in violation of the law under existing statutes, and those who obtain legal employment in clinics are prohibited from engaging in direct treatment and can act only as consultants.

The following suggestions were collated from 1974 interviews with fourteen acupuncturists most of whom had had lengthy training in the Orient plus several years of practice (Chow 1975: 90–2). These acupuncturists found themselves in situations in which, under existing laws, they were excluded as medical practitioners, yet, at the same time, they were solicited as experts to train physicians or to participate in research activities. In 1984, a decade later, their comments still serve as an appropriate critique and evaluation of the status of the current practice of acupuncture in most US states.

– All who practice acupuncture should have training for a minimum of four years, with continued training while practicing.
– Acupuncturists should be able to practice independently with full recognition of their contributions to medical care and treatment.
– Methods currently being used to teach acupuncture in the US are inadequate: one time workshops and seminar 'crash' courses offer superficial information for physicians and lay people. The effect of this is to discredit the value of acupuncture and the Chinese healing arts.
– Training should encompass the traditional philosophy and theory.
– Acupuncturists should not have to work under physicians in private practice or clinics receiving assistants' pay for their services while the physician garners high professional fees.
– Scientific research in acupuncture should be conducted in order to determine its relation to western medicine. This research should be carried out by acupuncturists expert in the particular specialty under investigation. A pediatrician, for example, is not necessarily expert in cardiology, nor is an acupuncturist experienced in musculoskeletal problems necessarily competent in the treatment of deafness.
– A common vocabulary needs to be developed to facilitate discussion about Chinese medicine.
– Acupuncturists need to broaden their knowledge in some of the basics of diagnosis, and in the nerve system, anatomy, and

physiology as these areas are utilized and understood in western medicine.

– In the normal sequence of health care, acupuncture should be considered as a treatment of choice, i.e. the patient should have the right to select and the practitioner to prescribe.

– The public needs to understand that acupuncture is not a panacea. An experienced and responsible acupuncturist advocates the treatment of certain pathologies by western technology.

– There must be verification of training and experience for all acupuncturists, including Asians already in the US, or entering the US, in order to determine the validity of their claims of being qualified practitioners.

Joseph Needham, who has extensively investigated Chinese medicine thinks that acupuncture has suffered wide "misunderstandings" in the west, with regard particularly to its being interpreted as parapsychological or occult. Needham does not see acupuncture, among other Chinese therapies, as contradictory to western scientific medicine. Implicit in this is the potential tie-in between the contributions of western analytic and empirical work in individual physiological units and the "synthetic" Chinese approach which "relates biological events to the overall systemic laws of homeostasis, balance, and integration" (Kao 1979: 4).

Considering that medical care in our society is in a period of transition from acute care to preventive and ambulatory care, the concepts and methodologies of Chinese traditional medicine, if properly utilized can now begin to enhance our technological progress and provide an impetus toward a more universal medicine.

References

Capra, F. (1975) *The Tao of Physics*. New York: Bantam New Age Books.

Chow, E.P.Y. (1975) *Acupuncture: Its History and Its Educational Significance to Western Health Practices in the USA*. A PhD thesis in Education. Fielding Institute: Santa Barbara, California.

Chuang Tzu (1971) Trans. James Legge, arranged by C. Waltham. New York: Ace Books.

de Langre, J. (1971) *The First Book of DO-IN*; (1976) *The Second Book of DO-IN*; (1975) *The First Western DO-IN, Acupuncture and Shiatsu Atlas.* Magalia, California: Happiness Press.

Fung Yu-lan (1964) *A Short History of Chinese Philosophy.* New York: Macmillan.

Huard, P. and Ming Wong (1968) *Chinese Medicine.* Trans. B. Fielding. New York: McGraw-Hill World University Library.

Kao, F.F. (1979) China, Chinese Medicine, and the Chinese Medical System. In F.F. Kao, and J.J. Kao (eds) *Recent Advances in Acupuncture Research.* Garden City, New York: Institute for Advanced Research in Asian Science and Medicine.

Kurland, H. (1977) *Quick Headache Relief Without Drugs.* New York: Morrow.

Li, C.P. (1975) A New Medical Trend in China. *American Journal of Chinese* Medicine 3(3): 213–21.

Lu, Gwei-Djen and Needham, J. (1980) *Celestial Lancets: A History and Rationale of Acupuncture and Moxa.* London: Cambridge University Press.

Mahdihassan (1982) The Term Chhi: Its Past and Present Significance. *Comparative Medicine East and West* 6(4): 272–76.

Namikoshi, T. (1973) *Shiatsu: Japanese Finger Pressure Therapy.* San Francisco: Japan Publications.

——(1974) *Shiatsu Therapy: Theory and Practice.* San Francisco: Japan Publications.

Palos, S. (1972) *The Chinese Art of Healing.* New York: Bantam Books.

Shanghai College of Traditional Medicine (1981) *Acupuncture: A Comprehensive Text.* Trans. J. O'Connor and D. Bensky (eds) Chicago: Eastland Press.

Traditional Acupuncture Foundation (1981) *A Summary of Current Acupuncture Legislation.*

Veith, I. (1970) *Huang Ti Nei Ching Su Wen: The Yellow Emperor's Classic of Internal Medicine.* Berkeley, California: University of California Press.

Wallnöfer, H. and Rottauscher, A. von (1972) *Chinese Folk Medicine.* Trans. M. Palinedo. New York: New American Library.

Wei, Ling Y. (1979a) Scientific Advance in Acupuncture. In F.J. Kao and J.F. Kao (eds) *Recent Advances in Acupuncture Research.* Garden City, New York: Institute for Advanced Research in Asian Science and Medicine.

——(1979b) Theoretical Foundation of Chinese Medicine: A Modern Interpretation. In F.J. Kao and J.F. Kao (eds) *Recent Advances in Acupuncture Research.* Garden City, New York: Institute for Advanced Research in Asian Science and Medicine.

Zhuo Da-Hong (1982) Comparative Therapeutic Exercise: East and West. *Comparative Medicine East and West* 6(4): 263–71.

Five

Indigenous systems of healing: questions for professional, popular, and folk care

Arthur Kleinman

Introduction

Over the past twenty years, medical anthropologists and cross-cultural psychiatrists have greatly advanced our knowledge of indigenous healing systems: what they are, how they fit into a particular social context, how they compare to psychotherapy and biomedical health care, and what they tell us about the healing process generally (see Kleinman 1980 for an extensive list of references). In the past five years, field research has generated the first group of systematic outcome studies that begin to indicate how effective indigenous healing is, what kind of problems it appears to be more *and* less successful in treating, and that even suggest what kinds of toxicities it may at times produce (Finkler 1980, 1981; Ness 1980; Kleinman and Gale 1983; Salan and Maretzki 1983). Remarkably little of this work has been conducted in North American or Western European societies. Indeed, most of what we know about indigenous healing derives from studies conducted in non-western societies. The irony is that while most researchers of indigenous healing systems come from the west, we know relatively little about indigenous healing.

The social development literature of the past almost always took the point of view that as developing societies modernized and westernized, indigenous healing would wither on the vine, while biomedicine would blossom forth as a new growth that eventually would substitute fully for whatever indigenous practices previously flourished. This viewpoint, like so many others in social development, has turned out to be wrong. Not that biomedicine has not flourished in non-western societies – it usually has (see Carstairs 1983 for a rural exception); but indigenous healing in most developing societies has tenaciously persisted, sometimes even enjoying a period of major growth at the very time biomedicine in the same setting is rapidly expanding (Leslie 1976; Kleinman *et al.* 1978).

If one thinks about it, this empirical reality is not surprising. For in North America, Western Europe, and Japan – the developed world – indigenous healing has never ceased to exist. In certain forms – e.g. religious healing, non-biomedical holistic health practices, the health food movement, spas and water cures (especially in Europe), non-biomedical healing professions (traditional East Asian medicine in Japan, chiropractic in North America, homoeopathy in Europe) – it has enjoyed periodic revivals, including, at the present time, a major one.

The thrust of this review will be to summarize what we have learned about indigenous healing and to see what that information can tell us about biomedicine and healing generally. The focus will be clinical, in as much as I am a clinician, and for the more important reason that arguably the chief contribution of the comparative study of healing is the light it focuses on the clinician's *work* and the therapeutic relationship.

Before we assess indigenous healing systems, however, we need to define first, what they are, and second, how they relate to biomedicine, on the one side, and self-care on the other. To accomplish this, I will present a model of health care systems that encompasses each of these domains of care. But at the outset I must raise a caution: indigenous healing, as we shall soon see, even in one local social setting, is a variety of things, not one thing. It is ludicrous to treat the many forms of indigenous healing – such as, Chinese medicine, Pentecostal exorcism, chiropractic, Balinese spirit mediumship, Haitian herbalism, psychic surgery in the Philippines, the health food movement, lay therapies of hundreds of kinds, and indigenous practice in hundreds of societies – as homogeneous. What we have learned about indigenous healing is knowledge about particular healing systems and healers in particular social contexts at particular times. This highly specific local knowledge can be (and in this chapter will be) synthesized. But the synthesis must be treated with great caution and sensitivity to enormous differences and distinctive levels of application. Much the same sort of meaning should attend our analyses of biomedicine, of psychotherapy and of self-care. Each is plural and highly diverse. Therefore when we discuss healing we need to specify which type of healing, which healers, in which setting, under what conditions, at what time. And when we generalize, as we must if we are to make cross-cultural sense of this vast subject, we need to be precise at what level of abstraction, with what qualifications, for what range of practices and practitioners our generalizations hold. To do otherwise is to court disaster, a courtship, in my opinion, consummated in most non-technical (and not a few technical) publications on this perennially fascinating but profoundly treacherous subject.

So why attempt at all to review comparative research on indigenous healing? The answer lies in the need to see healing in both its most distinctive and most similar forms if we are to determine what are its universal and culture-specific characteristics. For this very reason, cross-cultural research on indigenous healing is important not only for what it tells us about indigenous healing in our own society or for what contrasts can be drawn with biomedicine, but even more because through such studies alone are we able to see the broader processes and range of realities of which biomedicine and indigenous healing in America are particular instances. Frequently, psychotherapists and biomedical physicians write about indigenous healing from the standpoint of how it compares and contrasts with their discipline. In this chapter, I wish to do the opposite: what can we learn about biomedicine, self-care, indigenous healing and the clinical work of doctoring across the healing professions in our own society by viewing these activities within the integrating framework of cross-cultural studies of healing (Kleinman, Eisenberg, and Good 1978).

One model of the arenas in which health care of all kinds is delivered in society, a model based on a large body of cross-cultural research findings, will allow us to quickly define indigenous healing and disclose its relationships to other forms of healing.[1] *Figure 5.1* displays the three major arenas of care that constitute a local health care system: *popular, folk and professional.*

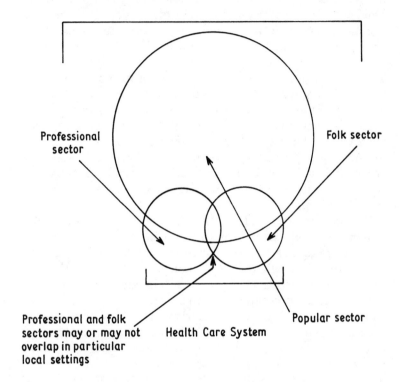

Figure 5.1 Local health care system: internal structure
Source: Modified from Kleinman (1980: 50).

Popular health care

If we examine what family members themselves perceive as sickness, then most health care can be shown to take place in the popular (or lay) health care sector (Demers *et al.* 1980;

Chrisman and Kleinman 1983). Here *illness* is first experienced, labeled, and treated by the individual (self-care), or more often by family members and other members of the social network. Popular health care practices are of a very wide variety and include health maintenance and curative interventions, of which the more commonly utilized are diet; special foods; local herbs and other traditional and contemporary indigenous medicines; massage; blistering and other manipulative techniques; exercise; changes in life style habits; use of biomedical drugs and apparatuses; symbolic interventions, ranging from charms and amulets to prayer, healing rites, and including various kinds of talking therapies. To the best of my knowledge, we possess no systematic studies of the effects of such "indigenous" treatments. But since in most societies most episodes of sickness perceived by family members never pass beyond the confines of the social network, laymen worldwide tend to regard these practices as potentially efficacious even though the better educated are not unaware that most symptoms treated in the kinship and friendship circle are minimal, self-limited, and readily normalized.

Of equal importance, the popular sector of care is where help-seeking decisions are made in the lay referral network regarding when to go to a particular practitioner for care, which practitioner to visit, whether to change practitioners or seek therapeutic alternatives, how long to remain in treatment, whether or not to comply with therapeutic recommendations, and how to assess outcome (Chrisman 1977; Chrisman and Kleinman 1983).

Indigenous healing, then, includes popular care in all its many forms. Since illness behavior is largely constituted in terms of the ethnomedical beliefs and norms of the popular sector, though it may sound paradoxical, the shaping of illness experience is a core therapeutic function of the popular sector (Kleinman 1980: 72–80). The placing of a sanctioned name on symptoms is an activity of paradigmatic social significance that is closely related to the processes of reproducing social order and meaning that Max Weber viewed as fundamental to every society. In most societies, counter to the views of healers, laymen regard the popular sector as the locus of responsibility for care. The most radical formulation of health care by consumer groups is not to legitimate indigenous healers, but to turn over to families sufficient knowledge and technical resources to better rationalize and provide more effective care in the popular sector. This is so clearly in the interest of cost containment, it would seem reasonable to assume, in spite of expectedly stiff professional resistance to empower laymen, that policy-makers will increasingly look upon such change as pertinent and practical. Yet the history of health care systems in the west suggests major structural and ideological barriers to such change, desirable as it may be, because it runs directly counter to the mainstream of modern social change that turns on professionalization.

Care in the popular sector is importantly influenced by economic, political, and cultural constraints. The popular sector of health care systems in developing societies tends to have greater access to biomedical drugs – frequently bought directly from a pharmacist without prescription and used at the family's or sick person's discretion. In western societies professionalization of health care has restricted popular access to drugs and to the knowledge and resources required to use them. But in recent years the health consumers movement can be viewed as a populist reassertion of popular sector prerogatives in health maintenance and health care.

Though we do not usually regard it as such, popular care is the most ubiquitous form of indigenous healing. There can be little doubt that the popular sector in North America and elsewhere in the west is at a serious disadvantage with respect to health care functions when compared with the popular sector in most developing societies. First, the much more limited social networks of the nuclear family in the west mean that the ability to mobilize social network, especially kinship, supports in the response to illness – a core therapeutic activity of the popular sector in more traditional societies – is lessened and with it are diminished traditional knowledge, and technical and personnel resources, to manage illness episodes. For example, Janzen (1978) has shown in Central African society that the kinship group forms a primary care "team" for managing illness episodes; a team that has had substantial experience both in practical care giving activities and in attending to the psychosocial tensions that are worsened or created by illness. Western societies, as we now well know, carry out many of the functions formerly rendered in the popular sector in bureaucratic settings. The critique of these tertiary role settings is that, not surprisingly, they fail to provide the sensitivity and skill in handling psychosocial issues that we associate with primary role social network settings. In this sense, indigenous family care is not care given to the family by a family doctor (which is really professional care), but care given by the family for its members. Perhaps no other cross-cultural insight into indigenous healing is more disturbing than the realization that the popular health care sector in the west has been seriously weakened by industrialization, urbanization, and the other components of modernization in North America and Western Europe over the last hundred years and more. For this means that the social buffers of stress, the major sources of interpersonal coping, natural systems for mobilizing personnel and funds to manage disability and death and dying, the chief system of transmitting and legitimating norms of how to experience and deal with illness are not available in the same way they are in the non-western world (and were in the west historically) as a core societal response to sickness. At present, we are witnessing a resurgence of the popular sector in the west, but while much is to be gained from strengthening lay care as an indigenous therapeutic system by increasing access to technical and knowledge resources now controlled by the professional sector so that health maintenance and simple, everyday primary care activities can be more effectively transferred to the family, there should be no romantic utopian expectation that we will see a revolutionary transformation of the popular sector of health care in the west. As Christopher Lasch (1977), Paul Starr (1983), and many other students of this subject have extensively documented, the determinants of change in the popular sector are long-term historical processes of economic and sociopolitical power that cannot be easily reversed and may even accelerate in the future.

Two final points about the popular sector. It is here obviously that over the long haul of biological and cultural evolution have materialized the sociosomatic and psychosomatic processes that embody a symbolic bridge between environment and physiology which mediates both certain contributions to disease causation (e.g. stress) and what might be called interior therapeutic reactions (e.g. autonomic nervous system, neuroendocrine and immunological responses to pathology;

Hahn and Kleinman 1983). Hence, it is an open question to what extent changes in the popular sector have affected (both positively and negatively) these processes. Could it be that the diseases of modernization – such as Type A personality and chronic cardiovascular disorder – represent at least in part fundamental changes in this biosocial bridge between popular sector and physiology? Here indigenous healing takes on entirely new significance as the health maintaining and pathology *damping* connections between social relations, meanings, and bodily processes.

The other point about the popular sector is more mundane, but no less important. There is a component of this sector, referred to as the commercial therapeutic sector, closely linked to the professional and folk sectors, which represents the big business side of health care (Fergusson 1981). There is practical gain associated with indigenous healing in even small-scale preliterate societies, and therefore it should not surprise us that economic interests are frequently inseparable from therapeutic ones. But the contemporary commercialization of indigenous healing in the popular and other sectors is still an awesome phenomenon. The health food movement is an impressive heterodox example of this, as is the more orthodox illustration of the pharmaceutical industry, but in fact an ideological patina of health concerns is to be found in the advertisements for many goods and services in the capitalist west. This commercial component of the popular and other health sectors should make us particularly wary of certain efforts to "reform" health care, like the current political pressure in America to make hospitals profit-making in the name of decreasing health care costs, or like the holistic health movement, which may (purposefully or inadvertently) further weaken the adaptive functions of lay care, and like the proverbial missionary go out to do "good", but end up doing "well" instead.

Professional health care

Mention of the professional sector conjures up images of biomedical facilities, but biomedicine is not the only component of the professional health care sector. In India, China, and Pakistan there are indigenous healing professions: Ayurvedia,

Chinese, and Yunani medicine respectively (Leslie 1976; Kleinman *et al*. 1978). In mid-nineteenth century America, eclectic and homoeopathic professions of medicine had their own schools and degree-granting procedures, and founded rival professional groups to biomedicine (Starr 1983). In contemporary America, osteopathy and chiropractic are alternative indigenous professions, with their own bureaucratic structure.

Indigenous healing, then, has a professional component. Although it is true that indigenous healing professions often are closer in their explanatory systems to the lay health culture, professionalization produces a *disease* (somatic, theoretical) rather than *illness* (psychosocial, experiential) orientation. For example, Ayurvedic practitioners and physicians of Chinese medicine redefine the illness problems their patients bring them in terms of their professions' somatic theories of etiology, pathophysiology, and treatment. This is the social construction of disease through specialist categories, out of the *illness* the patient and family bring to care (Kleinman 1982). This professional disease orientation is frequently associated with more formal relationships with patients, less time spent in explanatory interactions, and less attention given to psychosocial aspects of patient care than is found in non-professionalized folk healing systems, which appear to retain a closer relationship to popular cultural illness beliefs and treatment expectations. In my book, *Patients and Healers in the Context of Culture* (Kleinman 1980), I demonstrate these findings for Chinese medicine in Taiwan, and subsequent research in China convinces me it is true there as well. My reading of the medical anthropology literature suggests that it may be true of Ayurvedic medicine also. Nevertheless, while less close to native traditions than folk healing, indigenous healing professions are clearly closer to popular sector orientations, at least in non-western societies and likely also in the west, than is biomedicine.

Unlike the classical texts of the indigenous healing professions, which frequently pay substantial attention to psychosocial aspects of sickness and care, the actual practices of indigenous health professionals in the non-western world often tend to be technically oriented, somatopsychic rather than psychosomatic, and are concerned with curing disease more than with healing illness. At least this is the case in the day-to-day practice of traditional Chinese medicine (Kleinman 1980: 259–86). Having made this point, it is none the less the case that practitioners of indigenous healing professions, have been repeatedly described (by researchers and others) as more oriented to care of the whole patient than are their biomedical colleagues in the same kind of health care system. In Taiwan, practitioners of Chinese medicine spend more time with their patients and more time explaining to patients and answering their questions than do their biomedical colleagues (Kleinman 1980: 283–86).

In an important study in the United States, Kane and his colleagues (1974) showed that when faced with matched patients with low back pain, orthopedic surgeons and chiropractors had roughly the same outcome results, save that patients were much more satisfied with the care they received from chiropractors, who spent more time with them and whose personal characteristics seemed more supportive and concerned. This study not only buttresses the point I am making, but further suggests that self-selection and professional selection into indigenous healing professions may lead to a greater number of candidates in these professions who are primarily interested in the psychosocial aspects of care than is the case in biomedicine. Another contributing factor is professional training itself, which in indigenous professions like chiropractic, Ayurvedic medicine, and Chinese medicine appears to place greater importance on the doctor–patient relationship.

The lesson here is obvious and impressive: professionalization tends to distance practitioners from patients and to prioritize concern for disease ahead of interest in illness. Western-oriented biomedicine seems to be the more extreme example of this trend, perhaps because biomedical ideology and norms are more remote from (one almost wants to say estranged from) the life world of most patients. This is certainly the case in the non-western world; yet even here there is evidence of *indigenization* of biomedicine such that biomedical practice occurs in non-western societies within a framework that increasingly integrates local cultural expectations and behavior (Weisberg 1983).

These well supported generalizations to the side, it is worth puncturing some myths about indigenous professions. First, the actual practice of such professions is frequently quite distinctive from the classical ideology of the profession. Few Chinese physicians I have met or studied in Taiwan or China, for example, come up to that tradition's model of the classical scholar. Moreover, Chinese medicine and Ayurvedic medicine, as well as other indigenous healing professions, are modernizing, and have been for some time. Hence, there are substantial changes in the way the profession is practiced. In China, traditional Chinese medicine is increasingly practiced by professionals who combine biomedical and Chinese medical training. These professionals often replace the theory of Chinese medicine with that of biomedicine. They may use western methods and instruments, like stethoscope and blood pressure cuff, and may prescribe both Chinese medicines and biomedical drugs. This "integrated" practice infuriates philologists and historians who are students of the classical tradition and who are appalled by impurities brought into that tradition. But I suspect such borrowings and adoptions have occurred throughout the history of all professions and are a sign of a living, changing tradition in contradistinction to an historical artifact.

In Chinese and Indian societies as well as in the west, indigenous healing professions do not possess the high status of biomedicine. Many of these borrowings – white coats, stethoscopes, laboratory apparatuses, etc. – are somewhat crude attempts at status enhancement by copying the symbolic trappings of biomedicine. The obverse phenomenon is the travel of westerners, who practice acupuncture, Chinese medicine, or other non-western healing traditions in their own society, to the indigenous society to study with a "true scholar" or guru. This journey often seems to be more a quest for legitimation and obtaining symbolic power from a culturally sanctioned "source," especially when the sojourner does not bother to learn the indigenous language, than a real effort at acquiring indigenous training.

Folk health care

The folk sector of the health care system comprises non-professional, non-bureaucratized "specialists." Students of folk healing often divide this sector into sacred and secular subsectors, to indicate its roots in both religious (e.g. shamanism) and empirical (e.g. herbalism, bone setting, systems of massage and martial exercise) traditions. This sector is what is usually meant by the term indigenous healing. Today it is possible to speak of modern and traditional forms of folk healing. The examples I have just given are traditional folk healing traditions in Taiwan. In American folk healing, herbalists, Evangelical healers, Christian Science healers, and indigenous ethnic folk practitioners (i.e. Mexican–American curanderos, Puerto Rican spiritists, Haitian voodoo healers, Navaho singers) comprise the traditional folk subsector. Whereas so-called lay therapists (hypnotists, family therapists, pastoral counselors, polarity therapists, sex therapists, and practitioners of a bewildering variety of modern healing techniques) and health food advisors, for example, represent modern forms of folk healing. McGuire (1983) enumerated 130 kinds of folk healing in a middle-class suburb of New York City.

Folk healers are usually individual practitioners who practice outside institutional settings either in their homes or in the homes of patients. Sometimes folk healing is part-time and so widely shared a tradition that it blends into the popular health care sector. At other times folk healers seek to form a sanctioned healing profession and take on the bureaucratic trappings of a profession. Few folk healing practices are licensed, save for certain kinds of lay therapists in certain states, most are quasi-legal, and in some places they are illegal (e.g. shamans in China). Snow (1974) has shown that in urban black communities, some religious folk healers are frankly charlatans out to bilk an unsuspecting public. This is also part of the tradition of the snake oil salesman and medicine show proprietors of an early era. The numerous Asian healers who tour the United States, sometimes with an entourage of devotees which includes American business school graduates organizing their promotional campaigns, as well as the approximately 1,000,000 lay therapists who compete with mental health professionals for clients (Beitman and Eisdorfer 1983), indicate that there are substantial amounts of money to be made in indigenous healing.

Decades of anthropological and psychiatric studies of folk healers have produced an immense literature. But only in the last five years or so have we received the results of systematic outcome studies of patients treated by folk healers (Dobkin de Rios 1981; Finkler 1980, 1981; Ness 1980; Kleinman and Gale 1983; Salan and Maretzki 1983). These studies document three things: that folk healers are frequently effective, that there are limits to their efficacy, and that, while toxicities of folk healing are infrequent, they do occur. Much speculation has suggested that folk healers are principally effective because of their ability to foster psychosocial change (i.e. reintegrate social bonds, remoralize depressed patients and key family members, assuage tense and problem-generating interpersonal and even, at times, community relationships, and provide cultural and personal meaning for the illness experience). And these assertions appear like a tired refrain again and again in the ethnographic literature. Yet Kleinman and Gale (1983) found that folk healers in Taiwan were not more skilled at treating illness problems (the life problems associated with sickness) than their biomedical colleagues. They learned, furthermore, that both groups of healers did better with acute and self-limited disorders, somewhat less well with chronic illness conditions, and were specifically ineffective and unhelpful in the treatment of difficult psychosocial concomitants of medical disorders and most notably, of mental illness. This finding from a more comprehensive survey goes counter to a large body of anecdotal impression and ethnographic description, including the clinical observations of Kleinman himself (1980), who earlier had argued from a small series of cases, that Taiwanese folk healers were effective in healing illness experience, and relatively ineffective in treating disease. The Kleinman and Gale report suggests the efficacy of folk healers at least in Taiwan may be a great deal more complicated and less easy to interpret. Since this paper is one of the first systematic outcome studies comparing biomedical and indigenous healing it should make readers wonder whether the anthropological literature is perhaps implicitly biased in favor of indigenous healers just as the clinical literature often seems implicity biased against folk and popular health care practices.

Interestingly, although more than 75 per cent of matched patients in both groups improved, a surprising finding was that biomedical physicians had somewhat higher rates of successful outcome and patient satisfaction than did shamans. This finding needs to be replicated before generalizations can be made, but in the absence of pertinent studies we are authorized to lend it some heuristic significance.

These data upset our usual stereotypes of physicians and sacred folk healers, suggesting that the actual on-the-ground situation is more uncertain and variable. Researchers studying folk healing in non-western settings have at times engaged in a romantic, reverse ethnocentrism that has tended to exaggerate the therapeutic successes of folk healers and to use folk healing as a hammer with which to hit biomedicine on the head. In recent years, researchers have been less inclined to overstate the case for folk healers and have attempted to provide a more balanced portrayal of their strengths and weaknesses. I have studied dozens of folk healers in Taiwan. Few were as insensitive to patients' needs as were tertiary care physicians I studied in that society and in my own. But also few were as skilled in rigorously identifying and systematically responding to psychosocial and psychiatric problems as were biomedical residents I have trained in primary care fields and psychiatry.

It is clear that we are witnessing a major change in the way primary care internal medicine and especially family medicine are practiced in North America. Perhaps in response to consumer demands, and much less probably owing to the alleged strengths of indigenous healers, the primary care wing of biomedicine has increasingly legitimated psychosocial problems as an appropriate focus for care. Whether the funding sources of care will support such psychosocially sophisticated practices in biomedical clinics is another question. But biomedicine is as heterogeneous as is indigenous healing, and is undergoing a great if not greater change.

What, then, have we learned from studies of indigenous folk healing? First, in spite of controversy and uncertainty, we can say that early studies indicate most patients who attend indigenous healers get better after treatment (Finkler 1980, 1981; Ness 1980; Kleinman and Gale 1983; Salan and Maretzki, in press). More studies are needed, especially of indigenous healers in the west, to document what percentage of patients with different kind of disorders improve. At present, the best we can say is that most seem to improve who are suffering from acute self-limited disorders, and that many improve who suffer chronic disorders. But some afflicted with acute severe medical disorders (but not many) also do well. The findings for psychiatric disorders are more unclear. Psychoses, save short-lived reactive psychoses, do not seem to do well in indigenous care, but the literature on depression, anxiety, and other neurotic disorders can be read in two ways. Most of the literature, as I have already noted, suggests that it is precisely these disorders as well as psychosocial problems that are well handled by indigenous healers (see, for example, Leighton *et al.* 1968; Lambo 1969; Torrey 1972; Fabrega 1973; Frank 1974; Obeyesekere 1976; Reynolds 1976; Tambiah 1977; Janzen 1978; Sharon 1981; Dobkin de Rios 1981; Connor 1982, among many, many others). The few systematic outcome studies also indicate good outcome for certain problems: for example, acute stress-induced psychosocial and psychophysiological problems and mild acute neurotic disorders. But the tale for serious clinical depression, anxiety, and personality disorders has not yet been concluded. Further research is needed to settle the important disagreements over whether these problems do in fact have good outcome in indigenous practice. Less certain than outcome findings are data on the sources of efficacy in indigenous healing: how is indigenous healing effective? Here, in spite of much speculation over what might be the biopsychosocial basis of therapeutic success, there is little to report that is well founded. There is no question that certain healers use biologically active drugs that induce pharmacological effects in patients. There is even more impressive evidence of much more widespread sociosomatic and psychophysiological effects of social support, counseling, and ritual experiences, but the specific mechanisms by which these effects are brought about await sophisticated measurements of psychosocial and biological interaction. Although limbic system, endogenous opiate like substances, autonomic nervous system, neuro-endocrine system, immunological system, and cardiovascular and gastrointestinal systems appear to be involved in these responses, it is still not known how these systems are affected.

Enough is known, however, to puncture utopian hopes for cures for cancer or for the other major sources of mortality in the west. As each new traditional therapy is assessed in biomedicine, expectations become more realistic. Thousands of traditional medicines touted for efficacy against cancer have been tested by the National Cancer Institute and found to be ineffective. Acupuncture, originally claimed to be effective for a wide spectrum of disorders, has had efficacy demonstrated only for some kinds of pain. Yet these more limited effects on morbidity should not go unesteemed. Healing is a tinkering trade, difficult enough in the best of times and downright frustrating with great regularity, it needs all the proven friends and real help it can get.

Any effective treatment must have side effects (even the placebo provides nocebo effects: Hahn and Kleinman 1983). Some traditional Chinese medicines contain powerful biomedical drugs (e.g. prednisone), usually not labeled, whose side effects are well known, but Americans have complained of side effects with acupuncture (pain, hematomas, and local infection) and even with ginseng (e.g. gastrointestinal complaints). Some insensitive and less psychosocially skilled folk healers have angered patients and families (Kleinman 1980), some have caused delay in receiving potentially effective biomedical treatment for patients with biomedically treatable disorders who have worsened under indigenous therapy (Harwood 1981; Lin, Kleinman, and Lin 1982). Since we are just beginning to hear of studies of the toxicity of psychotherapy in the west, it is not realistic to expect similar data on the toxicities of ritual healing, but this should become an important topic for future research. All in all, then, there are many fewer reports of serious toxicities with indigenous healing, but some do occur.

Second, a very large amount of descriptive data (ethnographic, survey, and clinical) supports a set of categories for comparing folk healing *and* other therapeutic relationships (Kleinman 1980: 207–08):

1 Institutional setting (i.e. specific location in a given health care system's sectors and subsectors).
2 Characteristics of the interpersonal interaction:
   (a) *Number* of participants (i.e. in non-western societies few indigenous folk healing or other healing relationships are dyadic, most involve key members of social network as well as the patient, and this is also true of traditional ethnic groups in the west).
   (b) *Time* coordinates (i.e. whether it is *episodic* or *continuous*, folk healing may be either; the expected average

length of treatment; the amount of time spent in each transaction; the time spent in communicating or in explaining).

(c) *Quality* of the relationship (i.e. whether it is *formal* or *informal* with respect to etiquette, type of social role – primary, secondary, tertiary, emotional distance, restricted or elaborated communicative code, nature of transference and countertransference; whether it is *integrated* into or *divorced* from everyday life experience and ongoing daily activities).

(d) *Attitudes* of the participants (i.e. how practitioners and patients view each other, including respect, dependence, paternalism, fear, and particularly if they hold mutually ambivalent views of the other).

3 Idiom of communication:

(a) *Mode* (i.e. psychological, mechanistic, somatic, psychosomatic, sociological, spiritual, moral, naturalistic, etc. *idioms of distress*).

(b) *Explanatory models* (i.e. shared, openly expressed, tacit, or conflicting; whether the EMS are drawn from single, unified belief systems or fragmented, pluralistic ones).

4 Clinical reality (the way a "case" and treatment regimen are socially constructed in the doctor–patient transaction):

(a) *Sacred* or *secular*,

(b) *Disease-oriented* or *illness-oriented*,

(c) *Symbolic* or *instrumental interventions*,

(d) *Therapeutic expectations* (i.e. concerning etiquette treatment style, therapeutic objectives, and whether these are shared or discrepant).

(e) Perceived *locus of responsibility* for care (the individual patient, family, community, or practitioner).

5 Therapeutic stages and mechanisms:

(a) *Tripartite organization*:

(i) Sanctioning an illness problem and naming its cause in culturally appropriate symbolic terms;

(ii) Manipulating the cause symbolically to effect cultural cure; practical advice and help with illness problems; identifying social network problems and contributing to their resolution; providing personal support for patient and key family members to reduce anxiety and remoralize depressed individuals;

providing role models of efficacy; and using medicinal agents, physical manipulation and other somatic therapies;

(iii) Sanctioning a positive outcome: proclaiming and authorizing cure in cultural, social, and psychophysiological terms.

(b) *Mechanisms of change* (i.e. catharsis, insight, psychophysiological, social persuasion, conditioning, etc.).

(c) *Managing outcome* (i.e. handling chronicity, recurrence, treatment failure, disability, death and dying; enforcing adherence; negotiating termination and discrepant assessments of efficacy and satisfaction).

For each indigenous healer, or any healer for that matter, we can describe and compare his or her practices in terms of these clinically relevant categories. Of course, we could add other categories too to fill out the social context such as the demographics of healer and clients; healer's personal biography; history of entrance into healing (for sacred healers this often involves a "call to cure" via personal illness experience); training; and therapeutic experience (years in practice, number of clients treated, types of problems seen, reputation, etc.). But the categories I have outlined are the essential areas to determine the nature of the therapeutic relationship and healing practices. Reading through this list, I think it will strike readers that even indigenous healers of the same kind practicing in the same setting may differ somewhat on this analytic grid. Hence the crucial recognition is emphasized that indigenous healers are pluralistic. One can generalize about shamans in Taiwan, herbalists in Haiti, spiritualists in Puerto Rico or New York, curanderos in Los Angeles, or Navaho singers, but the more detailed the description the greater the differences, differences based on particularities of practice, setting, personality of healer, clientele, and particular cases. This awareness of differences even within the same type of indigenous practice should prevent the superficial generalizations and trite, mischievous comparisons that abound when indigenous healers are discussed (Torrey 1972). It is the awareness of differences that makes it difficult to answer the questions: Is indigenous healing effective? (Yes, but . . .). Dangerous? (Not often, but . . .). Can it be integrated with biomedicine? (Sometimes, but . . .). The answers require specificity of which healers? In what context? Healing what kinds of problems? Now that the World Health Organisation has promoted the integration of indigenous folk healers in many developing societies, we can expect that in future more substantial data may be available to answer these questions.

Coreil (1983) has made the interesting point that indigenous healers like biomedical practitioners can be grouped into primary care practitioners (midwives, bone-setters, herbalists) and tertiary care practitioners (voodoo specialists). She presents data from Haiti to show that in assessing which indigenous healers are more integrable with primary care and which with tertiary care specialists like psychiatrists, it is essential that this distinction be made.

Before concluding our description of the indigenous components of health care systems, it needs to be emphasized that these practices and systems do not stand on their own, but are embedded in historically derived *contexts* of cultural meanings, social norms, and political and economic power. These contexts have much to do with the salience of folk healing and its relationships to biomedicine. Starr (1983) discloses how the social transformation of American medicine narrowed the space occupied by folk practitioners and usurped activities previously the prerogative of popular health care. Similarly, the current interest in holistic medicine and alternative healing systems seems best explained as an historically derived populist movement that is perhaps rightly viewed by the medical establishment as anti-professional. Whether this movement is the last bright flicker of a candle about to go out, or represents a major reorientation of how health care will be delivered in our society is a question that the history of the 1980s and 1990s will answer.

This sociopolitical movement has increased the salience of self-care, popular care generally, and of alternative practitioners. It has stimulated two distinctive responses within the house of professional medicine: a negative reaction from the centers of high technology care and the planning and organization of health delivery systems; and the holistic, or perhaps better, the biopsychosocial movement in primary care (Engel 1977, Smith and Kleinman 1983, Kleinman 1983). Indeed family medicine might be seen as an attempt to reorient the values of biomedicine in keeping with this broad-based populist movement and the professional critique it has generated. Family medicine has become an advocate for viewing illness in the broad context of family and social network, health maintenance and prevention as authorized clinical goals, stress and behavior as core foci of the physician's task, counseling as a legitimate practice of the medical practitioner, and psychiatry and behavioral science as essential components of the physician's training (see contributions in Taylor 1983 and in *Journal of Family Practice*). Many of the same concerns, to a lesser but not insignificant degree, are surfacing in primary care internal medicine. Concern for women's issues in health is fairly wide spread in both fields and increasingly so in that former bastion of biomedical narrowness, obstetrics, and gynecology. In the last instance, the change in perspective can be seen to be an example of the re-education of their practitioners by women patients as well as by changing public opinion.

The response of family medicine, primary care internal medicine, nursing practice, and paramedical professionals might be seen as an attempt to transform biomedicine into a practice that includes certain aspects of indigenous healing that bring medicine into closer relationship with the popular health care sector.[2] Concern with improving clinical communication, attending more to psychosocial aspects of illness, recognizing ethnic influences on care, giving pregnant women wider choices in style, type, and location of delivery, and including advice on life style, exercise, diet, family relations, work, and even non-biomedical treatments is an example of this new indigenization of biomedicine. The tension within these fields – and in psychiatry – between this orientation and a resurgence of concern that a narrow biomedical model is needed or medicine will lose its intellectual rigor, scientific status, and professional identity is a sign that a major intraprofessional conflict is looming. History suggests that such a conflict is not resolved within a health profession itself but in terms of the wider context of the health care system as it reflects sociopolitical, economic, and cultural change in the societal context of care (Shryock 1969; Starr 1983). Within the perspective of the health care system, what we are witnessing is a realignment of the boundaries and relationships between the different sectors of health care in which popular sector and other forms of indigenous healing in

America are challenging the professional behemoth for greater control over health resources, decisions, and practice. Within the professional sector this challenge is in the form of "alternative medicine," and within biomedicine itself the primary care/tertiary care, medicine/nursing debates[3] are evidence of intraprofessional splits in response to this health system-wide period of change.

Conclusion

What are the practical policy and clinical implications of the perspective I have advanced in this chapter?

Policy-wise, I am concerned that no policy be advanced for enumerating, registering, and controlling non-professional indigenous healers in the United States or elsewhere, until more research is conducted that can determine if such activities would be beneficial or counterproductive to the nation's health care. I tend to think it would be potentially dangerous. First, because it might undermine a number of important indigenous practices – ethnic folk healers and popular care come immediately to mind – which seem to flourish in their present quasi-legal, unregulated status, and whose contribution is important precisely because it is non-professionalized and non-bureaucratized. Second, we know so little about indigenous folk healing in western society that ethnographic and survey research is needed to map this component of our local health care systems before we intervene. Attempts to regulate practice might well drive folk practitioners underground, as has happened in the past for certain kinds of practitioners. Once underground, quackery and downright criminality are readily attracted to healing. Third, the popular sector of care historically has been weakened in America by efforts to guide and rationalize its family-based and community-based functions. Professional definitions of "healthy" behaviors and "appropriate" self-care may raise suspicions that this may happen yet again, though only a fanatic would contend that no professional guidance is necessary to bring coherence to the immensely diverse and fragmented indigenous healing domain, where really effective practices may be lost in a sea of hyperbolic commercialism. Hence, my concern that even policy based on the best motives might yield unexpected and undesirable results: namely, bringing folk and popular sectors of care more under control of the biomedical profession. Having said this, however, I am also uneasy with the alternative, since those practices of folk healers that are potentially toxic or actually abusive of therapeutic powers should be controlled. The problem is how best to proceed. I favor local research, followed by community-wide debates about what is to be done, in which regulating indigenous healing practices is a final, community, not professional, step.

I strongly support the idea that the locus of responsibility for care rests with patients and their families, and that increased knowledge and technical resources should be made available to individuals and families to enable them to take over routine primary care activities now controlled by biomedicine. I recognize this is a radical and difficult step which in the short run could create more problems than it solves. But over the long haul this is surely the direction we must travel if we are to take seriously personal rights and social obligations in health care, and if we are to significantly contain cost increases in the health care system.

Control must be increased through existing and new regulatory devices over the rapidly expanding commercial health care component of health care system. It is one thing for health care to be organized like a big business, and something else for it to be practiced like a business. The latter could seriously distort clinical work and jeopardize psychosocially-oriented care. We are in desperate need of studies that assess the clinical reality constructed in for-profit medical institutions, and how it affects patient care decisions and clinical practices. There is every reason to be fearful of the corporate take over of American medicine. The interests of stockholders are likely to be very different from the interests of good patient care; for instance, the economics of technical interventions would demand that as many of these be employed in each case as possible to maximize financial gain, and simultaneously that psychosocial interventions, which may help the customer but would not financially benefit the provider, be decreased. This could lead to a horrendous situation in which medical ethics becomes no more than good business practice, the patient as a customer becomes an occasion to increase profits and decrease expenses, not deliver better care, and clinical judgment becomes distorted by commercial interest. What we already know about abuses of the commercialization of indigenous healing cross-culturally is enough to make anyone worry about this potentially very dangerous social change (Kleinman 1980: 203–10, Ferguson 1981; Salmon and Berliner 1980;). Cross-cultural studies of healing make clear that there are universal aspects of the healing process which may not be narrowly "cost effective" but may be crucial to personal and social life, which are vulnerable to abuse and distortion, and which require a unique moral framework (the therapeutic relationship) to be fully developed. The corporation's bottom-line is not the interest best suited to guide such a system, and we can hypothesize that it may create havoc with humane care.

Greater support needs to be given to primary care as the appropriate setting for training medical students, residents, and allied health professionals, and for providing psychosocially more sophisticated care. This means increasing the funding, curriculum time, and status for this part of academic and professional medicine. The primary care perspective necessitates a biopsychosocial approach within which personal, interpersonal, cultural dimensions of care receive prime attention. Primary care also requires an integration of social science with biomedical science concepts and methods to provide the knowledge base for the greater than 50 per cent of all medical visits that primarily turn on personal and interpersonal problems. This I regard as *the* great challenge for clinical science: to rework medicine's paradigm of clinical practice to make it more responsive to indigenous patient values, beliefs, and expectations.

This policy line leads directly to what I take to be the practical clinical benefits of studies of indigenous healing for clinical work. Physicians cannot (and even if they could, should not) become folk healers. But health professionals can learn from indigenous healing (1) how to reorient its priorities to serve humane patient care; (2) that clinical care besides serving the utilitarian function of *disease* also must attend to the moral function of *illness*; (3) that social relations, personal meaning, and cultural values are universal modifiers of healing cross-culturally and must be legitimated in professional care; (4) that the care practiced in professional facilities today is only one component of a greater health care system, of which health professionals are *not* the locus of responsibility for treatment decisions and trajectories; and (5) that a willingness to take into account the perspectives of patient, family, and other practitioners within the wider health care system leads to both deeper understanding of disease–illness and better care. Not least of its lessons, consideration of indigenous healing, places *healing* (the work of doctoring, therapeutic relationships, patient care) at the very center of medical attention, a position it has not occupied either in biomedicine or in the policy debate on health care for some time.

Note

1 I use healing and health care as interchangeable terms in this chapter.
2 Some critics of "medicalization" might regard this development as an attempt on the part of professional biomedical institutions to engulf and incorporate threatening and competitive indigenous components of the other therapeutic sectors (Taussig 1980), but I do not agree with this conspiratorial theory. The fact simply is that biomedicine is strongly influenced by the cultural norms of the environing social structure, and in this instance it is responding (somewhat belatedly and haphazardly) to various elements of the cultural revolution of modernism that the west and much of the rest of the world has undergone over the past several decades (Carstairs 1983).
3 Nursing educators regard the care of illness a core nursing activity, and have agreed that this is the justification for social science becoming a corner stone of nursing science. Not insubstantial numbers of academic nurses are taking coursework or even advanced degrees in social science, in an attempt to raise the status of their profession and assert its autonomy by linking it to the behavioral sciences. Ironically, the marginal status of social science, in North America where the development is occurring at least, is probably improved to the same degree that nursing benefits from this symbiotic union. But there can be little doubt that social science will not become core to biomedicine until it is legitimated in the core health science – medicine.

References

Beitman, B. and Eisdorfer, C. (1983) The Demographics of American Psychotherapists. *American Journal of Psychotherapy* 37: 37–42.

Carstairs, G.M. (1983) *The Death of a Witch*. London: Hutchinson.

Chrisman, N. (1977) The Health Seeking Process. *Culture, Medicine and Psychiatry* 1: 351–78.

Chrisman, N. and Kleinman, A. (1983) Popular Health Care and Lay Referral Networks. In D. Mechanic (ed.) *Handbook of Health, Health Care, and Health Professions*. New York: The Free Press.

Connor, L. (1982) The Unbounded Self: Balinese Therapy in Theory and Practice. In A. Marsella and G. White (eds) *Cultural Conceptions of Mental Health and Therapy*. Dordrecht, Holland: D. Reidel.

Coreil, J. (1983) Parallel Structures in Professional and Folk Health Care: A Model Applied to Rural Haiti. *Culture Medicine and Psychiatry* 7: 131–51.

Demers, R. *et al.* (1980) An Exploration of the Depth and Dimensions of Illness Behavior. *Journal of Family Practice* 11: 1085–092.

Dobkin de Rios, M. (1981) Saladerra – A Culture-Bound Misfortune Syndrome in the Peruvian Amazon. *Culture, Medicine and Psychiatry* 5: 193–213.

Engel, G. (1977) The Need for a New Medical Model. *Science* 196: 129–36

Fabrega, H. and Silver, D. (1973) *Illness and Shamanistic Curing in Zinacantan: An Ethnomedical Analysis*. Standford: Stanford University Press.

Fergusson, A. (1981) Commercial Pharmaceutical Medicine and Medicalization: A Case Study from E1 Salvador. *Culture, Medicine and Psychiatry* 5: 105–34.

Finkler, K. (1980) Non-Medical Treatments and Their Outcomes. *Culture, Medicine and Psychiatry* 4: 271–310.

——(1981) Non-Medical Treatments and Their Outcomes. Part 2. *Culture, Medicine and Psychiatry* 5: 65–103.

Frank, J. (1974) *Persuasion and Healing*, 2nd edn. New York: Schocken.

Hahn, R. and Kleinman, A. (1983) Belief as Pathogen, Belief as Medicine. *Medical Anthropology Quarterly* 14(3): in press.

Harwood, A. (1981) In A. Harwood (ed.) *Ethnicity and Medical Care*. Cambridge, Mass.: Harvard University Press.

Janzen, J. (1978) *The Quest for Therapy in the Lower Zaire*. Berkeley: University of California.

Kane, R. L., Leymaster, C., Olsen, D., Wooley, F., and Fisher, F. (1974)

Manipulating the Patient: A Comparison of the Effectiveness of Physicians and Chiropractic Care. *Lancet* 1: 1333–336.

Kleinman, A. (1980) *Patients and Healers in the Context of Culture*. Berkeley: University of California Press.

——(1982) Neurasthenia and Depression. A Study of Somatization and Culture in China. *Culture, Medicine and Psychiatry* 6: 117–89.

——(1983) Cultural Meanings and Social Uses of Illness Behavior. *Journal of Family Medicine* 16: 539–45.

Kleinman, A. *et al.* (1978) *Culture and Healing in Asian Societies*. Cambridge, Mass.: Schenkman Publishing Company.

Kleinman, A., Eisenberg, L., and Good, B. (1978) Culture, Illness and Care. *Annals of Cultural Medicine* 88: 251–58.

Kleinman, A. and Gale, J. (1983) Patients Treated by Physicians and Folk Healers: A Comparative Outcome Study in Taiwan. *Culture, Medicine and Psychiatry* 6: 405–24.

Lambo, T. (1969) Traditional African Cultures and Western Medicines. In F. Poynter (ed.) *Medicine and Culture*. London: Wellcome Institute.

Lasch, C. (1977) *Haven in a Heartless World: The Family Besieged*. New York: Basic Books.

Leighton, A. *et al.* (1968) The Therapeutic Process in Cross-Cultural Perspective. *American Journal of Psychiatry* 124: 1171–183.

Leslie, C. (ed.) (1976) *Asian Medical Systems*. Berkeley: University of California Press.

Lin, K.M., Kleinman, A., and Lin, T.Y. (1982) Sociocultural Determinants of the Help-Seeking Behavior of Patients with Mental Illness. *The Journal of Nervous and Mental Disease* 170(2): 78–85.

McGuire, M. (1983) Words of Power: Personal Empowerment and Healing. *Culture, Medicine and Psychiatry* 7: 221–40.

Ness, R. (1980) The Impact of Indigenous Healing Activity, an Empirical Study of Two Fundamentalist Churches. *Social Science and Medicine* 14B: 167–80.

Obeyesekere, G. (1976) The Impact of Ayurvedic Ideas on the Culture and the Individual in Sri Lanka. In C. Leslie (ed.) *Asian Medical Systems* Berkeley: University of California Press.

Reynolds, D. (1976) *Morita Psychotherapy*. Berkeley: University of California Press.

Salan, R. and Maretzki, T. (1983) Mental Health Services and Traditional Healing in Indonesia. *Culture, Medicine and Psychiatry* 7: 377–412.

Salmon, J.W. and Berliner, H. (1980) Health Policy Implications of the Holistic Health Movement. *Journal of Health Politics, Policy and Law* 5(3): 535–53.

Sharon, D.G. (1981) *Wizard of the Four Winds*. New York: Free Press.

Shryock, R. (1969) *The Development of Modern Medicine*. New York: Hafner.

Smith, C.K. and Kleinman, A. (1983) Beyond the Biomedical Model. In R. Taylor (ed.) *Family Medicine*. New York: Springer-Verlag.

Snow, L. (1974) Folk Medical Beliefs and Their Implications for Care of Patients. *Annals of Internal Medicine* 81: 82–96.

Starr, P. (1983) *The Social Transformation of American Medicine*. New York: Basic Books.

Tambiah, S.J. (1977) The Cosmological and Performative Significance of a Thai Cult of Healing Through Meditation. *Culture, Medicine, and Psychiatry* 1: 97–132.

Taussig, M. (1980) Reification and the Consciousness of the Patient. *Social Science and Medicine* 14B: 3–13.

Taylor, R. (ed.) (1983) *Family Medicine*. New York: Springer-Verlag.

Torrey, E.F. (1972) *The Mind Game*. New York: Emerson-Hall.

Weisberg, D. (1983) Physicians' Private Clinics in a Northern Thai Town: The Social-Cultural Context of Biomedical Practice. Paper presented to the panel on Biomedicine in Asia, American Anthropological Association, Washington, DC.

Six

Psychic healing

Daniel J. Benor

Introduction

Healing in the forms of laying-on-of-hands and/or prayer and meditation for health has been practiced from the dawn of human civilization. Modern western medicine has looked askance at such practices, suspecting them of being no more than magical beliefs and superstitions, the products of "primitive" societies' wishes to cope with illnesses beyond the ken of indigenous healers. It is hypothesized by western medicine that such beliefs aid "primitive" people to feel less helpless in facing life-threatening diseases. At best, credit is given for efficacy of such efforts via suggestion (Frank 1961; Torrey 1972). Any successes reported under such treatments are attributed by western medicine to such mechanisms as "natural resistance" of the diseased, chance coincidence of treatments applied when the disease was waning of its own accord, "spontaneous remission," etc. Claims for efficacy of healing treatments are usually dismissed out of hand. Despite this rejection on the part of "modern" medicine, healers in non-industrialized and industrialized societies continue to treat a multitude of medical problems. Some of their results, witnessed repeatedly by reliable observers, are truly astounding (Casdorph 1976; Krippner and Villoldo 1976; Meek 1977; St Clair 1979).

Recent evidence demonstrates that criticisms and suspicions voiced by conventional medical critics are not justified. Scientifically controlled studies, utilizing untreated groups with similar conditions to those of healer-treated groups, have repeatedly demonstrated significant positive effects of healing. Exciting research is beginning to clarify the involved methods and mechanisms. A comprehensive review of these reports, along with research from related fields will shortly be available (Benor, in press).

Observation of other healers and personal study of some of these techniques have further convinced this author of their validity. Despite all of the above, there is a part of me that still gets goose-bumps and doubts my own senses in the presence of such healing. These healings appear to contradict most of my medical training and beliefs of "how the world ought to be." They force a re-evaluation of basic understanding and assumptions of nature and of one's place in the universe. It is thus not surprising that others have chosen to reject this evidence rather than to re-examine and possibly change those beliefs about the world which they have held since childhood, which have been reinforced through years of conventional western education, and which today continue to be supported by the conventional western medical establishment.

Principles

Psychic healing (called "healing" hereafter) refers to the beneficial influence of a person on another living thing (either animal or plant) by mechanisms which are beyond those recognized and accepted by conventional medicine. These mechanisms may include focused wishes, meditation, prayers, ritual practices, and the laying-on-of-hands. Some healers believe that in healing they are merely activating innate recuperative forces from within the healee. Other healers believe they are transferring their own energies to the healee. Others state they are merely acting as channels for healing energies from universally available cosmic sources. Many believe they must involve the intervention of spirits or of God. The latter commonly call themselves "spiritual healers."

Healers report that any illness can usually respond equally well to healing touch or to healing sent by them from a distance. They usually cannot predict which healee will be cured, nor do they keep clinical records to allow assessment of percentages of positive responses. They do not mind if healees are skeptical regarding the healer's powers, but say that when the healee doubts his own recuperative powers this is a detriment. A general consensus also indicates that a quiet, receptive, meditative state in the healee is conducive to a positive response and that anxiety can hinder the effects of healing.

Carefully controlled studies have repeatedly demonstrated significant effects of healing in plants (Grad 1967; Loehr 1969), yeast (Grad 1965; Barry 1968), bacterial (Nash 1982) and cancer cell (Snell 1980) cultures, and mice (Onetto and Elguin 1966; Watkins, Watkins, and Wells 1973; Grad 1967; Solfvin 1982). Controlled studies in humans demonstrated systolic blood pressure in hypertensives was reduced with distant healing (Miller 1980), and that anxiety in cardiac patients was reduced with on-the-body (Heidt 1979) and near-the-body (Quinn 1982) healing. Several studies investigate possible mechanisms for the effect of healing (Goodrich 1974; Krieger 1975; Miller 1977; Rauscher and Rubik 1983; Rein, in press; Smith 1972).

Numerous clinical anecdotal reports attesting to the efficacy of some healers' work are available (Worrall and Worrall 1965; Spraggett 1970; Turner 1974; Cassoli 1981; Vilenskaya 1981). Some more serious reports describe systematic observations of healers (Leuret and Bon 1957; West 1957; Strauch 1963; Turner 1969a–d; Rose 1971; Casdorph 1976). These provide helpful hints as to how healing might work, but are not as reliable as the controlled studies and are open to alternative explanations. A few books review and discuss healing from a variety of views (Krippner and Villoldo 1976; Meek 1977 and Benor, in press). Thorough reviews and discussions of psychic surgery are also available (Stelter 1976; Meek 1977; Benor, in press).

Healing is not a panacea for all ills. It works in some cases but not in others (Strauch 1963; Turner 1969a, 1969c). Why this is so and which cases are more likely to respond are questions yet to be answered.

History

Healing has been recorded through the ages in all parts of the world from as early times as records exist. Today invariably shamans ("medicine men") are found in all non-industrial societies (Eliade 1970; Harner 1980). From this observation we can deduce that such shamans almost certainly practiced in pre-recorded times as well. Earliest records from China, India, Assyria, Egypt, and elsewhere are replete with tales of healings, as are the Old and New Testaments (Meek 1977). Early Christian church records report occasional miraculous healings and the body's ability to produce unusual physical states such as stigmata (Thurston 1952). In the Middle Ages, European monarchs were alleged to possess healing powers and the royal laying-on-of-hands was a recognized social institution (Bloch 1973).

During these earlier centuries western concepts of health and illness were intimately tied to forces of nature via concepts of humoral influences (earth, air, fire, water) and to higher spiritual realms via religious influences. Healing by means that were not mechanistic was therefore not an alien concept. Primitive surgery and minimally effective pharmacopoeias were the only mechanical and chemical means available for amelioration of injury and illness. Healing was thus able to find a much more prominent place in non-industrial societies.

With the European Renaissance, the dominant world views shifted and new notions about the human being altered concepts of health and illness. Descartes proposed that mind was separate from body, purely the product of brain. According to this new theoretical supposition, mind could only know itself and could not affect the body. Coinciding with the Industrial Revolution, this led to an infatuation with mechanistic manipulations of the environment (including in it the human body), and an eschewing of non-material and spiritual concepts which were denigrated as "unscientific" (Pierrakos 1976; Meek 1977; Dossey 1983).

With the advent of modern medicine, including enhanced abilities to diagnose and treat disease, western views of illness have become even more firmly rooted in mechanistic concepts. Modern medicine teaches that every disease must have a cause which is either congenital (genetic), infectious, metabolic (hormonal or enzymatic), toxic, traumatic, neoplastic (cancerous), degenerative, or psychosomatic (due to emotional trauma). Except in the latter instance (discussed later) treatment is usually disease-specific: infections receive antibiotics; metabolic disorders are handled with hormones; cancers are given surgery, chemotherapy, and radiation; and diseases with no known cures are given palliative therapy, with the hopeful expectation that further research will find more suitable means to treat them. With such successes in so many areas of medicine by application of tangible therapeutic agents, non-physical, unmechanistic healing by prayer or touch seems likely to be a mere placebo. Only in the past few decades have controlled studies demonstrated that healing produces results beyond what can be explained by conventional western scientific thinking.

Distinctions between healing and modern conventional medicine

Healing is grounded in a broad holistic view of humankind. It presumes that the healer can bring about physical changes in the healee without mechanical or chemical manipulations of the healee's body. Touch may be used, but only to make contact with the healee. That is, massage and manipulations of the body are not generally used in healing. At first glance this might seem like a fantastic claim that would hardly be more than superstitious. Many health practitioners have commented on the comforting nature of human touch. Mothers "kiss away the pain" of their children. Doctors and nurses routinely touch patients as an important part of their bedside manner. It would thus seem that touch alone might reassure or relax the healee enough to account for some of the results (Frank 1957; Montague 1971; Barnett 1972). However, the controlled studies referred to above lead us to consider healers' claims more seriously and to look beyond superficial explanations.

Several theories may (individually or collectively) explain healing. The connection between body and mind was again "rediscovered" by western psychology and psychiatry only in the last few decades. Psychosomatic medicine is now a well studied field (though a sizeable portion of the medical community remains ignorant of its extent, if not also of its existence). Numerous and pervasive connections between mind and body have been demonstrated. Emotions, thoughts, and psychological conditioning of conscious and unconscious nature have been shown to produce neuro-hormonal changes in many organ systems and may even lead to physical illness. Ulcers and asthma are among the better known ailments of this type. Various treatments of psychotherapeutic nature have also been developed to help cope with such problems, including many varieties of psychotherapy (Fromm-Reichmann 1950; Greenson 1967; Janov 1970; Ferber, Mendelsohn, and Napier 1972), hypnosis (and other variations on the theme of suggestion) (Barber 1961; Frank 1961), desensitization (Wolpe 1958), biofeedback (Green and Green 1977, Brown 1979), bio-energetics (Lowen 1975), rolfing (Rolf 1977), visualization (Assagioli 1965; Desoille 1966; Samuels and Samuels 1975; Simonton, Matthews-Simonton, and Creighton 1980) and others. Thus many avenues are demonstrated as potentials for physical self-healing via mental and emotional mechanisms with the assistance of therapists. That is, a person has the potential via acts of will, conscious and unconscious learning and/or conditioning, and psychotherapeutic treatments to alter his or her physical condition. The psychotherapeutic changes are presumed to provide corrective emotional experiences and/or relearning of improved habits, self-concepts and the like. The mechanisms in such changes are initiated with intellectual, social, and emotional interventions on the part of the psychotherapist, based on verbal and/or body-language communication. Their physical effects are presumably brought about by alterations in central and autonomic nervous systems as well as in the endocrine glands (Green and Green 1977; Brown 1979), but possibly due to neurohumoral changes within the nervous system as well.

These psychosomatic mechanisms alone may in some cases explain part of the effects of healing. The healer may be something of a psychotherapist. In listening to the healee's history and in promising a possible cure the healer may relieve anxiety, provide reassurance and even suggest away symptoms, as can be done with hypnosis. Reducing anxiety and tension alone may produce very beneficial physical effects.

It is clear, however, that more is involved in healing than

suggestion. Suggestion cannot explain the significant results of healing on bacteria, yeast, or animals. It also cannot explain certain anecdotal reports such as the following (which hint that currently accepted western paradigms for explaining such phenomena are inadequate):

1 Healers often diagnose the healees' physical conditions without any prior acquaintance with the healees and without performing a physical examination in any recognized fashion by modern medical standards. This may be done in distant healing (Westlake 1973; Safonov 1981) as well as in touch healing (MacManaway with Turcan 1983). They may report that they "just know" what is wrong, that they sense this as visual imagery or tactile imagery (during on-the-body or near-the-body healing), or that spirits tell them the diagnosis. They may often accurately name diseases and describe symptoms in terminology they do not intellectually comprehend (Sugrue 1970).

An actual case history may help to illustrate such diagnostic abilities. A woman described to me how she came to a healer for advice about her husband who was hospitalized because of severe abdominal pains and fever which had lasted several weeks. He had undergone laboratory and X-ray examinations and consultation with several specialists without arriving at a diagnosis. His physician had set a time later that day to meet with consulting physicians to discuss the advisability of immediate exploratory abdominal surgery, the only procedure as yet not implemented. The healer, at a distance of many miles from the patient and without any direct contact with him, diagnosed a viral condition and predicted the physicians would recommend the operation. The healer emphatically advised that the patient delay his decision for two days, as he foresaw that the symptoms would spontaneously clear up by then. The patient followed this advice. Though initially the attending physician was upset at the delay, all were relieved when the condition resolved spontaneously, without surgical intervention.

At first glance such reports may seem like coincidental guesses. I have seen and heard enough of them, some with incredibly accurate details, to be convinced that many are probably far more than guesses, almost certainly in the

"paranormal" range of occurrence. Scientific research is still
needed to establish this more firmly.

2 People receiving healing often report sensations of heat,
cold, tingling, or colors during the treatments (Turner 1969
a-c; MacManaway with Turcan 1983). This is so regardless
of whether it is a touch or distant healing and regardless of
the distance between healer and healee, which can range
from inches to thousands of miles. Most commonly these
sensations are noted at the sites where bodily dysfunction is
present, but sometimes they may be noted elsewhere as
well. Healers also often report such sensations, especially
heat and tingling in their hands during touch or near-the-
body healings.

3 Joyce Goodrich, a psychologist who teaches healing, did her
doctoral dissertation on the ability of healees to report sensations which were related to distant healing (Goodrich 1974).
She demonstrated in a controlled study that it is possible for
independent judges to identify with a high degree of significance when healers were or were not doing distant healing,
by the subjective reports of the healees.

4 A healer named Oszkar Estebany, whose abilities as a healer
were clearly demonstrated in several of the above mentioned
experiments (Grad 1965; Smith 1972), reports that when he
holds objects in his hands they can take on healing properties
(personal communication 1982). He has deliberately used
letters, cotton, and water as media to convey his healing to
people who were far away and in need of healing. Such people
report they sense heat emanating from the materials he
"impregnates." I, too, have felt such a heat when I touched a
letter from Mr Estebany.

How can we explain such anecdotes and observations? They
seem to indicate that far more than suggestion is at work!

Extrasensory perception (ESP) and psychokinesis (PK)

These provide possible partial explanations for some of these
reports. Experiments have demonstrated beyond reasonable
doubt (Rhine 1970, 1976; Murphy 1970; Nash 1978) the existence of telepathy (mind to mind communication), clairvoyance, or psychometry (knowing information directly from an

object, without sensory cues), precognition (knowing the future) and PK (mind influencing matter). These so-called "psi" powers could account for many aspects of healing.

These most carefully researched findings have been known for decades. Studies demonstrating the existence of psi phenomena have been performed repeatedly, with greater attention to meticulous methodology and to statistical analyses than in a large portion of studies in psychology, psychiatry, and medicine. The conclusions they lead to are unsettling. They indicate that it is possible under certain limited conditions (which are as yet poorly understood) to read another person's mind; to know certain information about objects without sensory access to those objects; to know ahead of time what is to occur in the future; and to influence objects in the environment directly through acts of mind, without physical manipulations of the objects. It is not surprising that conventional scientists have been slow and hesitant to accept these findings, despite the inclusion of the Parapsychological Association in the American Association for the Advancement of Science in 1969.

The mechanisms for functioning of psi powers are not described acceptably for the scientific community. The greatest impediment to their acceptance has been the inconsistency of the appearance of the psi phenomena. This has made it difficult to perform repeatable experiments. Some go so far as to assert that all psi experiments must be in error (Hansel 1966; Alcock 1981). These critics rely most heavily on the assumption that some experimental techniques must have been flawed to produce the reported results. This assumption cannot be supported in a vast number of meticulously performed studies (Hyman 1982).

A further impediment to their acceptance is that psi events appear to require postulation of forces as yet not identified. This makes the conventional scientist most uncomfortable! Modern science would like to believe that extensions of currently identified forces and energies will ultimately explain all aspects of our universe. In contrast with this view, it is fascinating to read expositions of physicists which seem to point to a convergence of modern physics with mysticism (Capra 1975; Zukav 1979) and to see discussions of a need for paradigm shifts in order to make sense of our world (Bohm 1980).

As psi mechanisms are not yet clear, we cannot ultimately

explain healing by saying it is a psi effect. It does help, however, to see that psi type knowledge of and manipulation of physical conditions is supported by a body of research evidence from parapsychology.

Healers could make diagnoses via any single ESP mode or combination thereof, such as: telepathic information obtained from the mind of the healee, from the mind of an investigator of the healer who knows this information, or from the healee's physical condition; and/or precognitive information of diagnoses yet to be made. Healers could then bring about changes in the healees' bodies directly, via psychokinesis (mind over matter).

Further possible mechanisms to explain healing

These can be found in recent research indicating the probable existence of energy fields surrounding all living things. These fields are postulated to play a role in organizing and/or controlling the growth and physiological functioning of living things (Ravitz 1962, 1970; Burr 1972; Becker and Marino 1982). It can then be hypothesized that healers may bring about healings through interaction(s) of their own energy fields with those of the healee. Alternatively, healers may use PK directly to influence the healee's field. Through telepathy they may also indirectly activate the healee to influence his own field and/or body.

Less well-defined possible mechanisms for healing

These are based on healers' subjective reports regarding what they do to bring about a healing. Many use prayers, incantations, fasts, trance states, etc. In western terms, healers seem universally to enter a meditative type of altered state of consciousness (Tart 1975) when they are healing (Cade and Cox-head 1978). At the same time they feel a dispassionate love for the healee and a sense of ''being one with'' the healee and with the ''All'' (LeShan 1974). This has led to speculation that healing involves other dimensions of reality, where physical changes may be brought about by mechanisms only comprehended in terms or laws applying to those realities (LeShan 1974, 1976). In everyday, sensory-based perception, most people can only partially and imperfectly comprehend such processes. Similar explanations apply for the intervention of spirits and/or God, through whose agencies many healers believe the healings occur (Sanford 1949; Worrall and Worrall 1965; Chapman 1978; St Clair 1979). Much further work is needed to clarify which, if any, of the above mechanisms singly or in combination are actually required in healing and which are only superstitious trappings of the healers' belief systems and cultures.

We can clearly see that far more is involved in health and disease than the physical and chemical homeostasis addressed by conventional medicine. The fact that scientific investigations have not yet fully explored these mechanisms should not limit attempts to recognize and understand these phenomena. As a result of such studies, healing techniques can be better understood and applied and the conventional medical paradigm can be appropriately altered too. Though there is no full explanation as yet of how aspirin works, people certainly enjoy its benefits.

The precise understanding of interpersonal and self-healing through such proposed mechanisms should be on the forefront of research, very much indicated by the numerous clinical reports and initial controlled investigations in healing. To ignore these reports denies patients the choice of an effective adjunct to present therapies. If, as some skeptical scientists maintain, these alleged phenomena represent mistaken perceptions or beliefs, they should be exposed as such. Saying that they are not worth studying because our present understanding of medicine has no available explanation for their existence is like saying that the Darwinian theory of evolution cannot be worth studying because it is not consistent with Biblical teachings.

Learning to heal

Healing can be learned. It seems that most people have some healing abilities but that (as in most fields of human endeavor) there are those with greater and lesser natural gifts in this area.

In America several well established courses in healing are

available. Dolores Krieger together with Dora Kunz, a healer, have established a course which appears to be having the most impact in America. It is geared primarily for nurses and has inspired a number of doctoral dissertations on healing at NYU where Dr Krieger teaches (Krieger 1979). Joyce Goodrich, a psychologist who works with Dr Lawrence LeShan, teaches courses in distant healing (Goodrich 1978). Other more informal courses are offered by various healers, but I am not aware of any which are as firmly grounded in a scientific research orientation as the above. Without such grounding, it is hard to know whether students are being taught actual healing methods or mere rituals which are no more than placebos. Abundant evidence attests to the likelihood of the latter possibility when no measures are taken to assure otherwise (Beecher 1955; Shapiro 1960, 1971).

It is these more serious efforts which have begun to give healing a more respected place alongside other proven therapeutic modalities and to serve as models for future development of a therapeutic modality which promises to provide a most valuable addition to our methods of diagnosing and treating illness.

Healing in the United Kingdom

Healing has received greater recognition in Great Britain due primarily to the work of a dedicated group of healers. They organized British healers so that the public has a measure of assurance regarding the legitimacy of a member's claims to actually be a healer. These include: The National Federation of Spiritual Healers, the Spiritualist National Union Churches and Guild of Spiritualist Healers, the Atlanteans, the British Alliance of Healing Associations, the Maitreya School of Healing, the Spiritualist Association of Great Britain, and the World Federation of Healing.

Healers in England have also obtained governmental approval to practice in National Health Service hospitals at the request of either the patient or of his or her physician.

Though the majority of British physicians still do not accept healing (this impression is from informal, word-of-mouth surveys of healers and researchers), most generally do not object to the adjunctive assistance of a healer. As the British National Health System compensates physicians without regard to the number of patient visits, it is advantageous to the physician even if a healer only spends time to listen to clients. This saves the physician much bother.

Further factors are probably also at play, once given the above situation. Many physicians, raised and educated in the western mechanistic model of medicine (not only in England), become annoyed when having to listen to clients' vague somatic complaints which are actually expressions of emotional tensions. They tend to view such people as detractors from the doctor's more important and intellectually satisfying mission of diagnosing and treating physical illness. Conventional, mechanistic medicine has come to focus far more on the disease that the patient has, rather than on the patient that has the disease (an approximate quote of William Osler, a prominent American physician of the last century, still largely unheeded today).

A peculiar double standard exists in the relations between many British physicians and healers. Though the healers' presence in hospitals is officially sanctioned, many physicians are loath to have it publicly known they consult with healers or refer patients to them. Yet in private they may not only avail themselves of healers' help with patients' problems, but may ask for healers to minister to their own ills. The existence of healing so stretches conventional credulity that physicians still fear the censure of those among their peers and the public who are skeptical or incredulous regarding the efficacy of healing. The tremendous advantage in the British system is that the patients who wish the aid of healers may openly request and obtain it.

The British Medical Association, the official voice for British physicians, is however hostile to healers. Thought not stating this directly, they do so by implication in their injunction against referrals of patients by physicians to osteopaths. The inference is that other alternative medical practitioners are likewise proscribed (MacManaway with Turcan 1983). However, the General Medical Council, a governmental body established to monitor the medical profession, does not recommend any limitations on alternative medical practitioners (Fulder and Monro 1981).

Other aspects of healing in England are interesting. Most

healers (again, estimated by informal, word-of-mouth survey) believe that much of their work is achieved through the interventions of spirits, who are the actual agents for the healing. In fact, they label their work as "spiritual healing."

In the UK (and in the rest of Europe as well) there is a greater willingness than in the US to accept a claim for therapeutic efficacy without firm, controlled (i.e. using comparison groups) experimental data. This may partially explain the less hostile reaction to healers, and certainly contributes to the rather lax (by medical standards) criteria for the registering of healers. For registration, healers need only present the testimony of several patients who claim they were healed.

Healing in the United States

In the US the picture is quite different. Healers are not organized in healer-licensed groups, are not recognized officially by law, and may even be prosecuted for practicing medicine without a license. The picture is complicated by the fact that each of the fifty states licenses medical practitioners of all specialties according to its own criteria. All have laws that prohibit the "practice of medicine" without license, applied to healers as well as to anyone who pretends to be a physician or other licensed professional.

The American Medical Association (AMA) is a very influential body in the US. It has been traditionally very conservative and protective of the medical practices of its members. It is largely through the legislative lobbying of the AMA that laws have been passed and maintained to restrict alternative medical practitioners. Within its own organization, the AMA has in the past actively discouraged its members from associating with or referring patients to chiropractors and other alternative health professionals. Its ethics code of 1957 stated: "A physician should practice a method of healing founded on a scientific basis, and he should not voluntarily associate professionally with anyone who violates this principle." This was interpreted to limit physicians from associating with alternative health professionals such as healers. In 1980, under pressure of multiple lawsuits by chiropractors for conspiring to prevent them from practicing, this code was changed. The current code permits consultation with other health professionals (Reinhold 1980). Thus the climate seems to be more conducive for the acceptance of healers and other alternative health professionals.

The American Holistic Medical Association (AHMA) was formed because changes in the AMA code of ethics have not produced immediate changes in traditional attitudes and restrictive practices. The AHMA established itself independently to promote alternative medical approaches. This group is attracting practitioners who encourage their patients to participate in health maintenance and in actively helping their bodies to cope with and recuperate from illness. Though these holistic approaches are clearly consonant with psychic healing, this organization, too, is chary of endorsing a therapy which may be viewed by the establishment as too unproven.

To increase the availability of alternative health practitioners, other steps have been initiated in several states. Recently a proposal to register "alternative" health practitioners was considered in California by the Board of Medical Quality Assurance (BMQA).

Registered practitioners would be permitted to provide any form of treatment except surgery, tissue penetration, prescribing dangerous drugs, instrumentation beyond superficial orifices, and use of ionizing radiation, which would continue to be restricted to physicians, according to a BMQA report that contained draft legislation to revise the current Medical Practice Act. (Lewis 1982)

This would enable the public to have a wider choice in treatments for their ills, beyond those provided by conventional medical practitioners. Healers, now liable to criminal prosecution for their activities, could practice openly. Californians are rather known for their tolerance of liberal and nonconventional views. It is such lay persons who appear to be pressuring for this legislation. The bulk of "alternative" practitioners themselves are not organized in any coherent political fashion. Few other states are likely to consider such changes along this line for some time, and the attempt in California has even been postponed.

The State of Nevada created a Homoeopathic Medical Board in 1983, in parallel with the existing conventional Nevada

Medical Society (Mayfield 1983). The Homoeopathic Board licenses Doctors of Medicine (MDs) and Doctors of Osteopathy (DOs) who pass a State examination in homoeopathy. This is not as broad a change as that proposed in California, as it applies only to MDs and DOs. Nevertheless, it is yet another step towards increasing the availability of alternative health practitioners.

Policy implications in the US are complex. The fact that healers have not gained greater recognition and standings in the United States is partly their own fault. Unlike in the UK, they have not organized themselves or established their own registration or licensing procedures. American healers have been more individualistic and apolitical. Rather than respond by organizing to confront and alter the restrictive atmosphere of the AMA and the legal system as have the healers in England, they have chosen to remain inconspicuous. Many remain isolated in their subcultures, fearful of attack by the establishment.

In part this reflects an aversion for exclusivity, from which healers themselves suffer at the hands of the established medical system. Healers hesitate to sit in judgment of each other, at least publicly or openly. In part it may also represent an honest approach to the subject of healing. It has been suggested, and available evidence somewhat indicates, that most people possess some healing abilities (Cuddon 1968; Krieger 1979). Combined with the great difficulty in defining and demonstrating what healing is and/or is not, this poses problems in establishing clearer criteria for testing healing ability and licensing healers.

To avoid prosecution under the various state laws (many of them differing in divers particulars from each other), healers have several alternative courses of action.

1 They may declare that their work is a form of prayer and therefore protected under the Constitutional guarantee for freedom of religion. To further legitimate this stance they may obtain ordination in any of a wide variety of churches, some well established and others less so. For many, this is a quite comfortable arrangement, as numerous religious denominations have institutionalized healing services, even to the inclusion of a laying-on-of-hands. Though in modern times this has been viewed as a symbolic ritual, in historical

perspective we have seen that this probably originated in actual psychic healing.

2 Healers may obtain training, licensing, and/or certification in some form of recognized therapy, including chiropractic, physical therapy, psychology, or alternatives such as massage, etc. This gives them license to "touch patients in a healing manner." This may actually yield fruitful blendings of several therapeutic modalities. It may or may not be mentioned to the client that more is being done than massage, depending on the healer's assessment of his client's openness to this. (On the other side of conventionality, many health professionals are probably doing healing already, without conscious awareness of this!)

3 Healers may declare their work openly to be psychic healing. In some states they cannot be prosecuted for this so long as they do not touch the client and so long as they do not advise the client to neglect known beneficial conventional treatments. An obvious example in the latter category would be the use of insulin in diabetes.

Medical economics plays a major part in the American picture, as it does in England. The private practice of medicine is rather lucrative and the training of its practitioners long, arduous, and expensive. Healers in America pose a potential threat to the incomes of physicians who are in greater numbers lately and under competition from a widening variety of practitioners. This is a motivating factor (in addition to the other factors mentioned in the British situation) in attempts to exclude healers and other alternative therapists from legitimization and from reimbursement within the health care system.

If healers were to form "professional" organizations in America, they would have to challenge the conventional medical paradigm, change existing laws in each of the fifty states, and fight for a share of contracting health care dollars. Objections against healers' practice within hospitals controlled by physicians may be insurmountable, and attention to related issues of practice and public acceptance would require major investments of monies and time. In addition, it would demand difficult emotional/intellectual reorientations on the parts of the healers and hospital staff and administration, in each case having to be achieved individually because it is hard to dictate to a private hospital who should be on its staff to treat its patients.

As in the current California proposals, some advocate immediate relaxation of restrictions on the practice of healers to increase the availability of this alternative mode of therapy (as well as of others), enabling many more patients to enjoy its benefits. This would be a serious mistake, in my opinion. For all its faults, modern medicine has still largely adhered to the principle of *primum non nocere* (first do no harm) and has at least established institutional mechanisms to evaluate the efficacy of its treatments and to test and assure the clinical acumen of its practitioners. In recent years medical practitioners have been required to update their professional skills through continuing medical education as a requirement for annual relicensing in some states and for maintenance of specialty membership. Healers and other health care practitioners should be required to establish similar standards and tests of competence prior to being certified or licensed. Without such requirements, anyone can claim to be a healer, and the public would be subject to treatment by practitioners of unknown quality, as well as to potential fraud and abuse.

Though considerable time and effort would be required, healers should be able to develop criteria for certifying themselves. Tests for healers' abilities could include:

1 Healers could demonstrate their abilities to diagnose illness in patients whose illness has not yet been diagnosed by conventional means (to preclude simple telepathic or clairvoyant impressions from established sources), with conventional medical evaluations later confirming the diagnoses.

2 Healers could demonstrate cases of successful treatment of medical conditions with results which conventional medicine would not produce, again with confirmation of conventional medical evaluation. This would preclude chance success based on suggestion, spontaneous waning of illness, etc. (Strauch 1963; Rose 1971; Casdorph 1976).

3 It may prove possible to establish correlations between healing abilities and some laboratory tests such as alterations in hydrogen bonding of water and crystallization of chemical solutions (Miller 1977), effects on enzymes (Smith

1972), effects on bacteria (Nash 1982; Rauscher and Rubik 1983), yeast (Grad 1965; Barry 1968) or cell culture growth (Onetto and Elguin 1966; Snell 1980). Such tests could then be used to screen for healing abilities.

4 Established healers might more rigorously test diagnostic and healing abilities of those who claim such talents. There are indications that consensual validation may be possible in some instances of healing, for instance via apparent changes in auras or rays which sensitives can observe around the bodies of healers and healees (Karagulla 1967; Schwarz 1980; Jeffries 1982).

Research to validate and implement many of these suggestions is sorely needed. Unfortunately, the conventional medical establishment has shunned and blocked research as much as it has tried to do the same with clinical practice of healing. It is unfortunate that funding for such research as well as forums in journals for publication of results of healing research have been severely limited. Hopefully this will be changed in the future.

Future prospects

The potentials inherent in psychic healing are enormous on medical, theoretical, philosophical, theological, psychological, and social levels.

Medical applications of healing include valuable additional dimensions for diagnosis and treatment of disease. These will not replace all conventional treatments, as only a portion of healers' diagnoses are accurate and only a fraction of those patients treated by healers respond with measurable physical changes. Healing should be another among many possible diagnostic and therapeutic modalities available. Because of its safety (there are no known negative effects from healing) it should probably be one of the first measures tried in all but dire surgical, cardiological, or biochemical emergencies. It can, in addition, be a most useful complement to conventional therapies even in emergencies. For instance, pain of many causes has responded extremely well to healing (Knowles 1954, 1956; Krieger 1979; Cassoli 1981). This alone can be a great boon, as pain medicines have troublesome side effects, including addiction.

Healing can also contribute to humanizing medical therapies, which have become increasingly compartmentalized, automated, and in other ways dehumanized. Healing views the person as a unitary organism. Both in healing treatments and in healing research, the interactions of healers with the conventional medical community would enhance the acceptance and utilization of holistic approaches.

At present there is more evidence from controlled studies to advance healing as a therapeutic modality than there is to support the efficacy of chiropractic or osteopathic manipulations. Hopefully the zeal of proponents of alternative therapies will not override the call for deliberate and cautious steps in certifying healers before they are sanctioned by social and legal agencies. Though rapidly legitimizing alternative therapists such as healers would have a short-term benefit of increasing their availability, it could too easily be a long-term detriment in leading to abuses of this license. Ultimately a backlash of rejection of the wheat with the chaff could ensue.

The future of public acceptance of healers is in some measure tied to that of other alternative health professionals. Laws and attitudes which affect one group will also affect others. It would seem that caution and careful thought is warranted in the official recognition of all alternative health modalities.

On theoretical levels healing challenges our understandings of the functioning of the human body, adding dimensions of comprehension that have eluded conventional medicine. Healing is said by healers to involve energy fields which surround and interpenetrate the physical body. This may help to elucidate mechanisms of the growth and maintenance of health, as well, perhaps, as explaining heretofore little understood treatments such as acupuncture. It may also help to explain the interactions of astrological events with events of living things on Earth, in that biological energy fields may be influenced by solar flares, gravitational fields of the moon and planets, and so on (Gauquelin 1969; Burr 1972).

On philosophical levels, healing challenges our mechanistic view of the world, suggesting additional dimensions for conceptualizing man's relation with the universe. On theological levels it may provide some scientific basis for comprehending prayer, spirits and God. On psychological and social levels, healing can contribute much towards an awareness of people's oneness with their environment. This begins with a heightening of individual healer and healee consciousnesses, which appears to be a part of much that occurs in healing (Sanford 1949; LeShan 1974, 1976). Once aware of one's pervasively intimate interconnectedness with each other, one often also becomes aware of one's interrelationship with every aspect of the universe. Ecological issues have an immediate impact, as the despoiling of the environment becomes a despoiling of that which is felt to be a part of one's self. Promotion of planetary cooperation rather than nuclear annihilation thus becomes a natural goal. Therefore, in a host of not-so-subtle ways, the understanding of healing and its integration with other Alternative medicines can contribute to the betterment of humankind – beyond the apparent miracles of more rapid recuperation from individual illness.

References

Alcock, J.E. (1981) *Parapsychology: Science or Magic?* New York: Pergamon Press.

Assagioli, R. (1965) *Psychosynthesis*. London: Turnstone.

Bandler, R. and Grinder, J. (1979) *Frogs into Princes: Neurolinguistic Programming*. Moab, Utah: Real People.

Barber, T.X. (1961) Physiological Effects of "Hypnosis." *Psychological Bulletin* 58: 390–419.

Barnett, K. (1972) A Theoretical Construct of the Concepts of Touch as They Relate to Nursing. *Nursing Research* 21(2): 102–10.

Barry, J. (1968) General and Comparative Study of the Psychokinetic Effect on a Fungus Culture. *Journal of Parapsychology* 32: 237–43.

Becker, R.O. and Marino, A.A. (1982) *Electromagnetism and Life*. Albany: State University of New York Press.

Beecher, H.K. (1955) The Powerful Placebo. *Journal of the American Medical Association* 159: 1602–606.

Benor, D.J. (in press) *The Psi of Relief: A Review of Research in Psychic Healing and Related Subjects*.

Bloch, M. (1973) *The Royal Touch: Sacred Monarchy and Scrofula in England and France* (trans. J.E. Anderson). Montreal: McGill-Queen's University Press.

Bohm, D. (1980) *Wholeness and the Implicate Order*. London: Routledge & Kegan Paul.

Brown, B.B. (1979) *New Mind, New Body*. New York: Bantam.

Burr, H. (1972) *Blueprint for Immortality*. London: Neville Spearman.

Cade, C.M. and Coxhead, N. (1978) *The Awakened Mind: Biofeedback and the Development of Higher States of Awareness*. New York: Delacorte Press/Eleanor Friede.

Capra, F. (1975) *The Tao of Physics*. Boulder, Colorado: Shambala.

Casdorph, H.R. (1976) *The Miracles*. Plainfield, NJ: Logos International.

Cassoli, P. (1981) The Healer: Problems, Methods and Results. *European Journal of Parapsychology* 4(1): 71–80.

Chapman, G. (as told by Roy Stemman) (1978) *Surgeon from Another World*. London: W.H. Allen.

Cuddon, E. (1968) The Relief of Pain by Laying on of Hands. *International Journal of Parapsychology* 10(1): 85–92.

Desoille, R. (1966) *The Directed Daydream*. New York: Psychosynthesis Research Foundation.

Dossey, L. (1983) *Space, Time and Medicine*. Boulder, Colorado: Shambala.

Eliade, M. (1970) *Shamanism: Archaic Techniques of Ecstasy* (trans. W. Trask) London: Routledge & Kegan Paul.

Ferber, A., Mendelsohn, M., and Napier, A. (eds) (1972) *The Book of Family Therapy*. New York: Science House.

Frank J. (1961) *Persuasion and Healing*. New York: Schocken.

Frank, L.K. (1957) Tactile Communication. *Genetic Psychological Monographs* 56: 211–51.

Fromm-Reichmann, F. (1950) *Principles of Intensive Psychotherapy*. Chicago: Phoenix/University of Chicago Press.

Fulder, S. and Monro, R. (1981) *The Status of Complementary Medicine in the United Kindom*. London: Threshold Foundation.

Gauquelin, M. (1969) *The Scientific Basis of Astrology* (trans. J. Hughes) New York: Stein & Day.

Goodrich, J. (1974) *Psychic Healing – A Pilot Study*. Doctoral dissertation, Yellow Springs, Ohio.

——(1978) The Psychic Healing Training and Research Project. In J.L. Fosshage and P. Olsen, *Healing: Implications for Psychotherapy*. New York: Human Sciences Press.

Grad, B. (1965) PK Effects on Fermentation of Yeast. *Proceedings of the Parapsychological Association* 2: 15–16.

——(1967) The Biological Effects of the "Laying on of Hands" on Animals and Plants: Implications for Biology. *Journal of the American Society for Psychical Research* 61(4): 286–305.

Green, E. and Green, A. (1977) *Beyond Biofeedback*. New York: Delta/Dell.

Greenson, R. (1967) *The Technique and Practice of Psychoanalysis*. New York: International University Press.

Hansel, C. (1966) *ESP: A Scientific Evaluation*. New York: Scribners.

Harner, M. (1980) *The Way of the Shaman*. New York: Bantam/ Harper & Row.

Heidt, P. (1979) *An Investigation of the Effect of Therapeutic Touch on the Anxiety of Hospitalized Patients*. New York University: Unpublished PhD Dissertation.

Hyman, R. (1982) Book Review of Alcock and others. *Parapsychology Review* 13(2): 26–7.

Janov, A. (1970) *The Primal Scream*. New York: Dell.

Jeffries, R.J. (1982) Psychical Research in China. *ARE Journal* 17(3): 93–105.

Karagulla, S. (1967) *Breakthrough to Creativity*. Santa Monica, CA: DeVorss.

Knowles, F.W. (1954) Some Investigations into Psychic Healing. *Journal of the American Society for Psychical Research* 48(1): 21–6.

——(1956) Psychic Healing in Organic Disease. *Journal of the American Society for Psychical Research* 50(3): 110–17.

Krieger, D. (1975) Therapeutic Touch: The Imprimatur of Nursing. *American Journal of Nursing* 7: 784–87.

——(1979) The Therapeutic Touch: *How to Use Your Hands to Help or Heal*. Englewood Cliffs, NJ: Prentice-Hall.

Krippner, S. and Villoldo, A. (1976) *The Realms of Healing*. Millbrae, CA: Celestial Arts.

LeShan, L. (1974) *The Medium, the Mystic and the Physicist: Toward a General Theory of the Paranormal*. New York: Ballantine.

——(1976) *Alternate Realities*. New York: Ballantine.

Leuret, F. and Bon, H. (1957) *Modern Miraculous Cures: A Documented Account of Miracles and Medicine in the Twentieth Century*. New York: Farrar, Straus & Cudahy.

Lewis, R. (1982) Lay Healer Registration Hearings Planned. *American Medical Association News* 3 December: 1, 18.

Loehr, F. (1969) *The Power of Prayer on Plants* New York: Signet.

Lowen, A. (1975) *Bioenergetics*. New York: Penguin.

MacManaway, B. with Turcan, J. (1983) *Healing: The Energy that can Restore Health*. Wellingborough, Northants, England: Thorsons.

Mayfield, C.K. (1983) The State of Nevada Establishes a Board of Homeopathic Medical Examiners. *Journal of Ultramolecular Medicine* 1(2): 7–9.

Meek, G.W. (1977) *Healers and the Healing Process*. Wheaton, Ilinois: Theosophical Publishing House.

Miller, R. (1977) Methods of Detecting and Measuring Healing Energies. In J. White and S Krippner *Future Science*. Garden City, New York: Anchor/Doubleday.

——(1980) *Study of Absent Psychic Healing in Hypertension*. Report from Holmes Research Foundation. Los Angeles, CA.

Montagu, A. (1971) *Touching: The Human Significance of Skin*. New York: Columbia University Press.

Murphy, B. (1970) *Challenge of Psychical Research: A Primer of Parapsychology*. New York: Harper Colophon.

Nash, C.B. (1978) *Science of Psi: ESP and PK*. Springfield, Illinois: C.C. Thomas.

——(1982) Psychokinetic Control of Bacterial Growth. *Journal of the Society for Psychical Research* 51: 217–21.

Onetto, B. and Elguin, G.H. (1966) Psychokinesis in Experimental Tumorgenesis. *Journal of Parapsychology* 30: 220.

Pierrakos, J.C. (1976) *Human Energy Systems Theory: History and New Growth Perspectives*. New York: Institute for the New Age of Man.

Quinn, J. (1982) *An Investigation of the Effect of Therapeutic Touch Without Physical Contact on State Anxiety of Hospitalized Cardiovascular Patients*. Unpublished PhD thesis, New York University.

Rauscher, E.A. and Rubik, B.A. (1983) Human Volitional Effects on a Model Bacterial System. *Psi Research* 2(1): 38–48.

Ravitz, L.J. (1962) History, Measurement, and Applicability of Periodic Changes in the Electromagnetic Field in Health and Disease. *Annual of the New York Academy of Science* 98: 1144–201.

——(1970) Electromagnetic Field Monitoring of Changing State Functions. *Journal of the American Society for Psychosomatic Dentistry and Medicine* 17(4): 119–29.

Rein, G. (in press) An Exosomatic Effect on Neurotransmitter Metabolism in Mice: A Pilot Study. *European Journal of Parapsychology*.

Reinhold, R. (1980) AMA, Facing Legal Pressures, Adopts Less Rigid Code For Doctors. *New York Times* 23 July: A1–A12.

Rhine, L.E. (1970) *Mind Over Matter*. New York: Collier.

——(1976) *ESP in Life and Lab: Tracing Hidden Channels*. New York: Macmillan.

Rolf, I. (1977) *Rolfing: The Integration of Human Structures*. Santa Monica, CA: Dennis-Landman.

Rose, L. (1971) *Faith Healing*. London: Penguin.

Safonov, V. (1981) Personal Experience in Psychic Diagnostics and Healing. In Larissa Vilenskaya (trans and ed) *Parapsychology in the USSR, Part III*. San Francisco: Washington Research Center.

St Clair, D. (1979) *Psychic Healers*. New York: Bantam/Doubleday.

Samuels, M. and Samuels, N. (1975) *Seeing With the Mind's Eye*. New York: Random House/Berkeley, CA: Bookworks.

Sanford, A. (1949) *The Healing Light*. St Paul, MN: Malcalester Park.

Schwarz, J. (1980) *Human Energy Systems*. New York: Dutton.

Shapiro, A.K. (1960) A Contribution to a History of the Placebo Effect. *Behavioral Science* 5(2): 109–35.

——(1971) Placebo Effects in Medicine, Psychotherapy, and Psychoanalysis. In A.E. Bergin and S.L. Garfield (eds) *Handbook of Psychotherapy and Behaviour Change: An Empirical Analysis*. New York: John Wiley.

Simonton, O.C., Matthews-Simonton, S., and Creighton, J.L. (1980) *Getting Well Again*. New York: Bantam.

Smith, J. (1972) Paranormal Effects on Enzyme Activity. *Human Dimensions* 1: 15–19.

Snell, F.W.J.J. (1980) PK Influence on Malignant Cell Growth. *Research Letter, University of Utrecht* 10: 19–27.

Solfvin, G.F. (1982) Psi Expectancy Effects in Psychic Healing Studies With Malarial Mice. *European Journal of Parapsychology* 4(2): 160–97.

Spraggett, A. (1970) *Kathryn Kuhlman: The Woman Who Believes in Miracles*. New York: World.

Stelter, A. (1976) *PSI Healing*. New York: Bantam.

Strauch, I. (1963) Medical Aspects of "Mental" Healing. *International Journal of Parapsychology* 5: 135–65.

Sugrue, T. (1970) *There Is a River*. New York: Dell.

Tart, C.T. (1975) *States of Consciousness*. New York: Dutton.

Thurston, H. (1952) *The Physical Phenomena of Mysticism*. London: Burns Oates.

Torrey, E.F. (1972) *The Mind Game: Witchdoctors and Psychiatrists*. New York: Bantam.

Turner, G. (1969a) What Power is Transmitted in Treatment? (Pt 1). *Two Worlds* (July): 199–201.

——(1969b) I Treated Plants, Not Patients (Pt 2). *Two Worlds* (August): 232–34.

——(1969c) Experiment in Absent Treatment (Pt 3). *Two Worlds* (Sept): 281–83.

——(1969d) Psychic Energy Is the Power of Life (Pt 4) *Two Worlds* (Oct): 302–303.

——(1974) *A Time to Heal: The Autobiography of an Extraordinary Healer*. London: Talmy, Franklin.

Vilenskaya, L. (1981) Psychoregulation and Psychic Healing. In *Parapsychology in the USSR Part I*. San Francisco: Washington Research Center.

Watkins, G.K., Watkins, A.M. and Wells, R.A. (1973) Further Studies on the Resuscitation of Anesthetized Mice. In W.G. Roll, R.L. Morris, and J.D. Morris (eds) *Research in Parapsychology 1972*. Metuchen, NJ: Scarecrow Press.

West D.J. (1957) *Eleven Lourdes Miracles*. London: Helix.

Westlake, A. (1973) *The Pattern of Health: A Search for a Greater Understanding of the Life Force in Health and Disease*. Berkeley, CA: Shambala.

Wolpe, J. (1958) *Psychotherapy by Reciprocal Inhibition*. Palo Alto, CA: Stanford University.

Worrall, A.A. and Worrall, O.N. (1965) *The Gift of Healing*. New York: Harper & Row.

Worrall, O. (1981) Presentation at Healing in Our Time Conference, Washington, DC.

Zukav, G. (1979) *The Dancing Wu Li Masters*. New York: William Morrow.

Seven

Alternative medicine and the
medical encounter in Britain
and the United States
Rosemary C.R. Taylor

"Alternative" forms of healing and new ideas about how to stay healthy appear to be flourishing in both the United States and Britain.[1] How exactly one defines alternative (or fringe, natural, traditional, supplementary) medicine, why it is enjoying this burst of attention, and whether it will continue to do so are questions which have absorbed practitioners and commentators alike in the last few years. Skirting the question of definition, the editors of collections on non-allopathic medicine (Hulke 1979; Stanway 1982) tend to list everything that sounds vaguely alternative, and employ different criteria for their choices. The list is always a long one: biofeedback, acupuncture, chiropractic, spiritual healing, homoeopathy, naturopathy, and less well-known therapies such as iridology, bioenergetics, rolfing, and radionics. Some attempts at categorization have also included parapsychology and occult practices (Salmon and Berliner 1980b), native American healing rituals (Halberstam 1976), the promotion of "wellness" through nutrition and healthful lifestyles (Holden 1978), and "back-to-basics medicine" – "a return to treating the whole person instead of only the disease'' (Walton 1979: 410).

Why this strange spectrum of therapies should command such interest in the last decade in two western industrialized nations, whose citizens up to that point appeared to have been mesmerized by the technological sophistication of modern medicine, is a puzzle which this paper tries to unravel. I shall argue that different forms of allegiance to various alternative medicines are best explained by considering the growing pressures on the conventional doctor–patient encounter in both countries, and the nature of the relationship between practitioner and client which an alternative system of healing offers.

The growth of alternative medicines: an ambiguous phenomenon

The evidence for the emergence or rediscovery of alternative medicine is sketchy, since many therapies are labeled unorthodox or alternative precisely because they do not possess standard licensing requirements, societies, boards, training, and examinations. Yet the figures that do exist indicate that interest in these different therapeutic systems and approaches to health and illness has definitely grown, and that their devotees – both practitioners and clients – have increased in number. In the United States, the Biofeedback Society of America, founded in 1968, now has 1,750 members (Rubin 1979); in 1980 it was estimated that more than 23,000 chiropractors were treating eight million Americans for a variety of conditions (Wardwell 1980); and about 2,000 American medical doctors (MDs) are said to be ''involved with'' acupuncture (Hassett 1980).

In Britain more than 86,000 people were out-patients at the six homoeopathic hospitals within the National Health Service (NHS) in 1977 (Stanway 1982: 157). Almost no one practiced acupuncture twenty years ago; now the number who have been through training courses is estimated at 750 (Eagle 1980), while a recent survey has found 160 physicians who are also acupuncturists, and an additional 758 ''lay'' acupuncturists, 508 of whom belong to the professional association (Fulder and Monro 1981). Hypnotherapy boasts an amazing 1,630 practitioners according to the same survey, which in 1981 found a total of 29,898 practitioners of various kinds of what the authors prefer to term "complementary medicine." Excluding healers (20,020), the total number of non-medically qualified therapists is put at 7,800 – 28 per cent of the total number of general medical practitioners (Fulder and Monro 1981:36).

The growth in various forms of alternative therapy led last year to the formation of the British Holistic Medical Association, to a series of articles on alternative medicine in *The Times* (West and Inglis 1983a, b, c), and to a leader in the same paper entitled "Physician, Heal Thyself" (10 August, 1983) which remarked on the number of people turning to alternative practitioners and called the medical profession to task for the failings in modern medicine that this movement must indicate. The flurry of letters which followed revealed that alternative healing is a subject of interest to the medical profession and laymen alike in Britain at the moment.

The extent of alternative medicine's resurgence can also be gauged in terms of its success in removing a variety of legal restrictions on its practice. In 1966 the American Medical Association (AMA) house of delegates issued a policy statement which labeled chiropractic "an unscientific cult whose practitioners lack the necessary training and background to diagnose and treat human disease" (Culliton and Waterfall 1979). During the 1970s, however, chiropractors managed to persuade a number of private health insurance companies to cover their services. In 1973 payment for chiropractic treatments was approved under the Medicare program, provided that the problems they claimed to cure – which chiropractors attribute to "subluxations" (misalignment of spinal vertebrae) – were demonstrable by X-ray. Encouraged by these victories, chiropractors in the United States brought lawsuits against several states in the mid-1970s alleging that the defendants (AMA, the American Hospital Association (AHA), several medical specialty societies, the national organization of osteopaths, county and state medical societies, and the state association of pathologists among others) conspired to restrain the trade of chiropractors, and attempted to monopolize health services by medical doctors. In December 1979, the AMA settled out of court a case in Pennsylvania, agreeing that individual specialists, including radiologists and clinical pathologists, but not the profession as a whole, could associate professionally with chiropractors, which meant in practice that they could take patients who were referred to them by chiropractors (Dunea 1979). The legal situation with regard to acupuncture is more confused, but in some states, such as Pennsylvania, any physician can practice acupuncture (Hassett 1980). New York and California now license non-physicians to do so as does Nevada, provided that the technician is supervised by a five-person board (Africano 1975).

In Britain, under law, sickness and death certificates can be supplied by any competent person; in practice local Department of Health and Social Security (DHSS) officers usually accept certificates only from medically qualified practitioners. Coroners on rare occasions have accepted death certificates from an "alternative" practitioner such as a herbalist. In 1978 the Medical Adviser to the Civil Service, in a letter to the chairman of the British Acupuncture Association, reaffirmed that any competent person might issue a sickness certificate. In 1980, the Minister of Health reprimanded both the DHSS office and the Medical Tribunal, an appeal body, for refusing to take osteopathic notes as seriously as notes from a doctor (Fulder and Monro 1981: 6). Bans on referrals were removed sooner and with less resistance than in the United States. In the 1970s the General Medical Council rescinded the ban on physicians referring patients to medically unqualified practitioners, if they have the necessary skill and on condition that the referring doctor is ultimately responsible for the patient. Homoeopathy is recognized by Act of Parliament although in practice this legal protection is not enough, critics argue, as the government refuses to reimburse NHS general practitioners for tuition and other expenses incurred in attending courses in this field because the Council for Postgraduate Medical Education has ruled that training in homoeopathy "is not of sufficient relevance to modern medical practice to warrant financial support for courses for GPs" (cited in Parliamentary Correspondent 1978: 166).

Alternative therapeutic systems, then, have gained adherents and a number of legal obstacles to their growth have been removed in the last two decades. Whether however, they share enough common characteristics to be classified as a unitary phenomenon, their recent popularity explicable in terms of similar causal factors and shared origins, is difficult to say. The use of terms such as "holistic medicine" or the "holistic health movement" reflects an assumption that they do, but holism on closer inspection may yield component parts animated by principles different enough to dispel the illusion of unity. Salmon and Berliner (1980b) include in the list of holistic therapies any system that holds "as a cardinal principle the notion of the fundamental and integral unity of the mind, the body and the spirit" (p. 198), recognizing, however, that the term "holistic" is applied by some enthusiasts to systems that do not meet this criterion. They get around the problem by calling such therapies "alternative forms of healing" while acknowledging that "their advocates may call them 'holistic' "(p. 198).

A common epistemological basis seems non-existent. The explanations of illness which underpin alternative medicines invoke causal factors that are different from those favored by the "bacteriological orthodoxy" of conventional medicine (Wallis and Morley 1976) but also very different from one another. Mistaken beliefs are the source of ill health, according to Dianetics and Christian Science, whereas acupuncture is supposed to liberate energy pathways and restore a balance in the relative amounts of Yin and Yang energy flowing through the body. Some alternative therapies choose one part of the body and claim that all complaints can be diagnosed by examining it, or treated by realigning or otherwise working with it. Chiropractic focuses on the spine; iridology is based on the assumption that each organ of the body is represented by an area in the iris and that all disease can be diagnosed by examining it; advocates of the Ingham technique believe that there is a direct reflex action between the nerve endings in the feet and the various organs of the body. Diagnosis is achieved by "reading" the sole and relief obtained by pressing or massaging the appropriate area of the foot. Other theories of alternative healing blame most forms of ill health on one harmful habit. Diet is singled out in several systems as the most powerful source of a host of problems – cancer, crib death, nervousness, and hypoglycemia – and the single most effective treatment for many others: heart disease, appendicitis, arthritis, and varicose veins (Rynearson 1974).

Training varies widely. Those who practice some forms of alternative or holistic therapy are required to undergo several years of formal schooling (chiropractic, homoeopathy), while others are accepted into the community of practitioners by virtue of their possession of a special gift of intuition or grace (certain kinds of spiritual healer). Alternative healing systems are also derived from diverse cultures and different historical periods. Some persist from the nineteenth century or have been rediscovered (homoeopathy and chiropractic); a few have been transplanted from the east (acupuncture, reflexology and yoga); others claim to be traditional or folk remedies which have always existed (herbalism) and some alternative therapies are of fairly recent origin (biofeedback, rolfing).

Defining and classifying alternative medicine, therefore, has proved a difficult task: as a plethora of alternative titles implies, the nature of a revived unconventional, holistic, or complementary medicine remains elusive (Eagle 1980). Recent attempts to define it have concentrated on enumerating the characteristics which alternative healing systems presumably share and which differentiate them, in turn, from orthodox, scientific or western medicine.

They are to be distinguished from mainstream medicine, first, by their emphasis on the "subjective experience of the patient" (Salmon and Berliner 1980b: 198) and their insistence that therapists should focus on "the person rather than just the disease" (Holden 1978: 1029). Scientific medicine, in contrast, was distinguished at its inception by the view that the human body was "a machine, just like any other," which required service in the same way as any other machine needing repairs (Berliner 1982: 171). Patients were then isolated and treated as "cases." Modern medicine, in consequence, requires its practitioners to be emotionally detached to some degree, to concentrate on the disease and to avoid being distracted by their patients' "unique personal feelings and experiences" (Kane *et al.* 1974, Salmon and Berliner 1980b: 198).

Orthodox medicine venerates the expert, in this view, whereas alternative systems insist that the patient has the capacity and, indeed, often the responsibility, to become and remain well. The doctor acts "only as teacher and facilitator" (Holden 1978: 1029). The relationship between practitioner and patient is essential to the healing process; confidence and trust are taken to be as important as pills and good surgical technique, while the medicine to which we have become

accustomed, say its critics, relies on magic bullets administered by harassed physicians who cannot distinguish us one
from another as we flow from waiting room to examining room
to billing office.

Practitioners of holistic medicine are concerned with more
than the simple absence of illness which, they argue, does not
constitute health; they see their task as encouraging "complete
wellness" (Halberstam 1976; Callan 1979; Sechrist 1979), in
contrast to orthodox medicine which is obsessed with sickness
and the rooting out of disease. The procedures and remedies in
the armamentarium of modern medicine are characterized as
"technological," aggressive, and sometimes harmful. For diseases such as cancer the cure often seems more horrifying and
disfiguring than the disease itself. Alternative remedies, on the
other hand, are said to be "natural" (Atkinson 1978), safer
(Twemlow and Chamberlin 1981; West and Inglis 1983a),and
noninvasive (Salmon and Berliner 1980a). And, finally, as the
costs of conventional medical care eat up 10 per cent of the
Gross National Product in America and even 6 per cent in
Britain, holistic medicine, "generally provided on an ambulatory basis for stress prevention," with its laying on of hands,
its distaste for ferocious surgical interventions, and its avoid-
ance of hospitals, must be cheaper (Salmon and Berliner 1980b:
200; Berliner and Salmon 1980: 141).

But do alternative healing systems and holistic approaches
share all these features? Hypnotherapy, which bypasses the
patient's conscious wishes to reach into his or her destructive
unconscious fears and tensions, surely does not accord the
patient the same central role in the healing process as, say,
Christian Science. Chiropractic maintains that only a qualified
expert can locate subluxations and unblock the flow of nerve
impulses. There seems to be little that is "natural" or
noninvasive about the acupuncturist's technique of sticking
needles into various parts of the anatomy. Some kinds of alternative specialists train in schools which do not look very different from medical schools, go into private practice and, when
their services are recognized as competitive with mainstream
medicine, their prices become competitive too (Rossman
1975).

In the end, then, what one can say about alternative medicine
in the 1980s is that it seems to be defined by all the things that

scientific or allopathic medicine is not, even though this claim, too, is disputed. "In all these senses," says Halberstam (1976) of the orientations that holistic approaches to healing presumably share – treating the individual as a whole, the refusal to consider mind and body as separable in disease, the emphasis on wellness and the role of the individual as self-healer – "good medicine has always been 'holistic' " (p. 24). Physicians favoring holism, argues Walton (1979), are simply advocating an "almost conservative philosophy of care that includes all of traditional medicine" (p. 1411). There is also no evidence yet as to whether clients of alternative practitioners view them as a supplement to conventional treatments or use them exclusively, as a genuine alternative.

The popularity of alternatives: a response to the failures of conventional medicine?

Despite their ill-defined and heterodox nature, a range of non-conventional therapies seem to have captured the popular imagination in Britain and the United States, and the question is why. I shall concentrate for the most part on the revival of alternative medicine in its narrowest sense – a range of therapeutic systems which have a clearly defined knowledge base and an epistemology which differs from that underlying allopathic therapies – rather than include the range of lay practices, self-help groups and self-care activities which also seem to be increasing, but which usually share a common framework of explanation with conventional medicine.

The reasons adduced for the growth in popularity of these ideas and practices are as various as the alternatives themselves. A change in the cultural mood is often held responsible. Avina and Schneiderman (1978), for example, attribute alternative medicine's appeal to "a rising 'disenchantment with modern science and a return to occultism' " (p. 369), because many of its inspirational philosophies have a mystical character, its remedies demand faith in magic and intuition. Some alarmed observers see the holistic health movement as linked to much more rapid social and cultural changes which have produced an eruption of volcanic proportions, "an uncontrolled nuclear reaction [of] hypothetical institutes for this, academies for that, organizations for integration of East and West, and advocates for touching, thinking, and trotting,'' argues Callan, which is ''fanned by the flames of the 'me,' self-centered, generation'' (Callan 1979: 1156). Holden (1978) claims that the ''virtual explosion of interest in alternative healing methods and systems'' has been produced by ''consumerism and the human potential movement'' (p. 1029) as well as by public disillusionment with conventional medicine.

A second line of argument sees medicine as a reflection of societal developments broader than cultural changes. Berliner has argued that all forms of medicine are used to restore people to productivity within a certain form of society and so ''each therapeutic mode is consistent with the forces and relations within the society that contains it'' (Berliner 1982: 163). He distinguishes four major stages in the transformation of the American economy and four ''modes of production of healing'' which accompanied those stages. The one we are currently leaving behind, which he calls scientific medicine, is ''an industrial mode of production in which medicine is practiced by competing individuals and begins to assume a commodity form'' (p. 163). He predicts that the emerging mode of medical production will follow a similar if not identical path to that of the industrial sector during the period that America achieved a monopoly-capitalist economy. It has not yet produced a fully developed therapeutic, but Berliner assumes that the latter will emphasize measures to reform the lifestyle of individuals (such as campaigns to prevent smoking), rather than remove environmental or occupational sources of ill health which would constrain new sources of productivity and profit in the economy.

A particular *Weltanschauung* accompanies a particular stage in the development of economic production; dominant ideas justify and reinforce the activities and objectives of those who control the means of production. Hence, ''scientific medicine was not only similar to industrial production, it also validated capitalist production norms . . . [and] tended to both legitimate and reflect the existing social order'' (Berliner 1982: 171). If alternative medicine were to flourish, according to this view, it must somehow reinforce the purposes and position of a dominant group. Berliner makes this argument about the alternative practices which emerged in the nineteenth century. Homoeopathy, when it was first introduced into the United States in the mid-1840s, represented a reaction to the accepted forms of healing – violent techniques such as blood-letting. It was also "a form of market segmentation" in that it appealed to the upper class "for whom it was a form of conspicuous consumption – paying for something that was nothing" (p. 166).

Brown views medicine as connected to the development of capitalism in an even more instrumental way: it is a "tool developed by members of the medical profession and the corporate class to serve their perceived needs" (Brown 1979: 3–4). These are the actors responsible for the demise of homoeopathy and other medical sects at the turn of the century, a development usually understood in terms of the increased efficacy of regular or scientific medicine. Instead,

> the campaign to win acceptance for scientific medicine struck a responsive cultural chord among the new technical and managerial groups associated with industrial capitalism and with the media they controlled. The campaign established a popular belief in the broad effectiveness of scientific medicine and, together with political action by elite medical reformers, undermined the medical sects that competed with the regular profession.   (Brown 1979: 91)

Alternative forms of healing can be allowed to flourish as long as they "resonate with ideological changes in the economy" (Berliner 1982: 164), but if they pose a threat to ruling groups they will be crushed.

The major problem with arguments which assume that alternative medicines are a fairly direct reflection of broad economic or cultural transformations is that they ignore the differences among therapeutic systems. They also overlook the fact that alternative therapies seem to have divergent appeals for different audiences. The social base of homoeopathy as a social movement has always been the upper class, in both Britain and the United States. In Britain it sometimes appears that this was the result of a historical accident: homoeopathy attracted the interest and patronage of a few aristocratic figures, a phenomenon which continues, as witnessed by the often quoted fact that one of the royal physicians is a homoeopath. But in the United States, too, homoeopathy still attracts clients who are more highly educated and of a higher social class than the population as a whole (Avina and Schneiderman 1978). The adherents of Christian Science appear to be drawn from the same social base – "business and professional people, well educated and highly literate" (Lee 1976). Chiropractic, in contrast, attracts patients who are disproportionately working class (Firman and Goldstein 1975; Cleary 1982). Healing ministries have appealed traditionally to the "abjectly" poor, and in the most recent period to blacks, Indians, Puerto Ricans, and poor whites (Harrell 1975; Lee 1976).

Even if one were to argue, as Berliner has done, that there are gaps in any dominant system of thought which allow alternative therapies to emerge, that the very rich can engage in alternative practices, the very poor have to, and the marginal groups – immigrants, counter-culture, and religious minorities – choose to so engage (private communication), the particular fascination which some therapies hold for specific groups or fractions of groups is never specified. The precise mechanism of attraction by which some people are drawn to alternative medicines as cultural moods shift and modes of production are transformed is obscure.

Most of the arguments about alternative medicine's recent success, however, explain it in much narrower terms: alternatives expand and contract in popularity in proportion to the successes and failures of conventional medicine (Inglis and West 1983: 6–12). Its rivals' new lease on life in both Britain and the United States has been generated by the growing problems with an older system of healing that can no longer be concealed. The chronic illnesses of cancer, heart disease, and stroke contribute to the larger part of mortality and morbidity in western industrialized societies; medicine seems to be making little headway with them, and even less with the intractable social problems of drug abuse, alcoholism, venereal disease, and obesity which make ordinary people's lives miserable. To sufferers from the chronic pain associated with back and neck injuries, arthritis and rheumatism, medicine also rarely offers relief. Such failures have led to a massive popular rejection of scientific medicine, hence the new following for alternative remedies.

The scientific breakthroughs, this interpretation continues, are now on the side of the alternatives. The endorphins, which were discovered in the mid-1970s, are natural chemicals found in the brain, similar in structure to opiates like heroin and morphine. They provide a scientific rationale for acupuncture's analgesic effects and perhaps for the operation of other therapies: they "work psychosomatically, the body obeying the mind through a broadcasting system emanating from the brain, whose transmission system is only gradually coming to be understood" (West and Inglis 1983a: 6). Testimonials and anecdotal evidence (Williams 1976; Eagle 1978; Romano 1980; West and Inglis 1983b: 6) seem to indicate, above all, that alternative therapies *work* in many cases. Just the hope that they might work is enough because everything else has failed; alternative medicine provides a last resort.

Modern medicine, according to its critics, has shortcomings other than mere lack of efficacy which may have driven patients to seek out alternative practitioners. Iatrogenic disease – the injuries which stem from medical interventions and drugs which are supposed to cure but in fact exacerbate the problem – is frequently cited as a reason for public disillusionment with medical advances (Eagle 1978: 31; Salmon and Berliner 1980a: 542; Inglis and West 1983: 8–9). Wallis and Morley (1976) argue that orthodox medical care is not readily available to large sections of the population and that, where this is so, marginal medical practice will emerge to fill the gap. Roebuck and Quan's study (1976) of health care practices in a small Mississippi town seems to provide some supporting evidence for this argument. The inhabitants who grew up in a period when conventional medicine did not always penetrate rural areas continued to use traditional remedies and voiced skepticism about scientific medicine. Practitioner utilization also varied by ethnicity although, again, it was largely the *older* blacks and whites who seemed to differ significantly from one another in their orientations towards medicine.

The deficiencies of conventional medicine, however, do not seem to explain in its entirety the phenomenon of the last two decades: the resurgence of alternative treatment methods. Orthopedists, for example, have rarely been able to offer total relief to all patients suffering from back injuries; why should such patients suddenly turn to alternative healers now? Medicine's therapeutic failures may explain some part of public disenchantment, but they do not explain the decision of some patients to try alternative therapies. Similarly, as numerous studies in the history of medicine have argued, the acceptance of a new therapeutic by the medical profession or the public is rarely due solely to its demonstrated efficacy (Parssinen 1979).

The rise in alternative therapies probably cannot be attributed to the cost and uneven distribution of modern medicine. First, these factors do not explain the *recent* renewal of interest in other healing systems; cost and access are enduring problems. Second, policy-makers who deal with health care in the 1980s perceive one of their most vexing problems to derive from the fact that consumers rarely feel the cost of the services they use because a large part of that cost is covered by third party payers. Alternative therapies, on the other hand, with a few exceptions such as chiropractors' services under well defined conditions, are covered neither by private insurance schemes in the United States nor by the NHS in Britain. Alternative medicine, if widely adopted, might well have a dampening effect on the overall level of health care costs, but to the individual consumer such services, for the time being, usually appear to be an added expense. It is hard to determine whether lack of conventional medical care drives people to see alternative practitioners. One of the few studies which attempted to gather more information about this issue found that in Muscatine, Iowa, a medically underserved rural area, chiropractors did not appear simply to "fill in" where conventional physicians were unavailable for primary care (Yesalis *et al.* 1980.)

This raises the question of whether the phenomenon is created by supply or demand. The number of people applying to train in various branches of alternative medicine has risen dramatically in the last decade (Wardwell 1980; West and Inglis 1983c). We could be witnessing an effort on the part of students, who face increasingly stiff competition to gain admission to medical schools, to forge alternative career paths. Or it may be that the willingness to turn to practitioners of another healing system varies according to the disease with which the patient is afflicted. We can speculate that cancer patients, whose disease has not been halted by conventional therapy, may be willing to try anything since they have little to lose, so that judging the general level of public interest in alternative medicine from the number of patients using laetrile would be misleading.

The origins of the followings that different alternative systems are able to command in various historical periods may turn out to be dissimilar. The healing ministries in the United

States, for example, were at their strongest during the 1950s and seem to have had little to do with the level of public confidence in conventional medicine. The prestige of the latter, in fact, had never been higher. It looked as though its new tools – chemical and antibiotic therapy – could eradicate the causes of many illnesses. The healing revival which occurred during the same period derived its support from a huge social and religious movement among the poor (Harrell 1975), whose institutional support was the small pentecostal churches after World War II. The movement's support declined in the late 1950s because of the loss of financial support which was largely due to the growing opposition on the part of the pentecostal churches. Fraud and extremism also played their part as did familiarity: "miracles became too commonplace, claims too unbelievable, prophets too available" (Harrell 1975: 7). But the independent revivalists found new paths to follow: the old healing ministries were replaced by a much broader charismatic revival within which healing "remained an important doctrinal – and promotional – plank" (p. 8).

Alternative medicine may have to be disaggregated into its component parts, therefore, if one is to come up with a convincing explanation for its recent success. Different therapies may have gained adherents for diverse reasons, not all of which may be expected to relate to developments within modern medicine. There is one feature of the latter, however, which does bear closer examination for its potential to explain both some part of the public disaffection with conventional medicine *and* the attraction of alternative therapies. According to numerous studies and commentaries, patients who turn to alternative healing systems apparently do not do so because they find new theories of disease causation persuasive (Avina and Schneiderman 1978). The one consistent theme (in addition to therapeutic failure) in consumers' responses and in observers' speculations is dissatisfaction with the *relationship* which obtains with conventional physicians (Firman and Goldstein 1975; Parker and Tupling 1977; Eagle 1978) and the attraction of a different kind of relationship with alternative practitioners. Homoeopathists turn out to spend more time with their patients than do conventional physicians, to devote meticulous attention to each sympton whatever its origin and to insist on the uniqueness of each person's symptoms (Avina and

Schneiderman 1978: 369). Chiropractors are differentiated from other physicians because of their "patient" orientation (White and Skipper 1971); natural therapists are considered to be superior to general practitioners at an interpersonal level (Parker and Tupling 1977).

Rosenberg has argued about therapeutics at the beginning of the nineteenth century that they were related to a broad cognitive system of explanation, on the one hand, and to "a patterned interaction between doctor and patient, one which evolves over centuries into a conventionalized social ritual" (Rosenberg 1979: 4), on the other. This is no less true of modern therapeutics. Like class, medical practice is, above all, a relationship; it cannot be described exclusively in terms of developments within medical science. It is not a mere reflection of changes in production which made certain kinds of medical knowledge ideologically consonant with a capitalist view of the world. Nor is it imposed by groups of doctors in those periods when they gain the leverage to realize their self-interested objectives. The rise and fall of different healing systems, I argue, is contingent in large part on the changing nature of the medical encounter. To understand the patterns in this relationship, one must look beyond physicians' organizations and motives which affect but do not encompass the fluid historical connection between healer and patient.

The demand for participation

Without romanticizing the relationship between doctor and patient or overlooking the hardships they endured in the early years of this century, it is safe to say that health care has grown from the provision of a personal service to the "delivery" by a complex industry of a vast array of products and benefits. In the context of this expansion, it became commonplace to draw parallels with other industries. It was assumed, for example, that the providers and managers of health care services would become aware of a deterioration in the quality of their product through mechanisms similar to those that alert the management of firms and other organizations: customers would stop buying the product or the organization would lose members (what Hirschman (1970) has called the "exit option"), or management would be subjected to complaints, either directly from dissatisfied customers or, with the emergence of a shared public concern, through the media (the "voice option").

Dissatisfaction with the nature of the medical encounter, however, is not so easily expressed or resolved. Until recent decades it was not a primary focus of concern. In the United States, with the consolidation of professional authority and the expansion of medicine's technological arsenal in the 1920s, few questions were raised about the quality of the relationship between doctors and patients; rather, the central problem in health care was defined as access: the wonders of medical science were not available equally to all consumers. After World War II, the state intervened with several solutions. The Hill–Burton Act provided more money for hospital construction; the National Institutes of Health (NIH) were established to ensure that the high quality of the product, medicine, would be maintained; and the introduction of Medicare and Medicaid in the 1960s was designed to allow the old and the poor to enjoy, with everyone else, the benefits of a progressively more impressive health care system. During Johnson's War on Poverty, critics asserted that perhaps the problems of access were more complex, that providers were not sensitive enough to the barriers to medical care (other than the simple cost of services) that poverty entailed: poor transportation, limited hours which ignored the problems of two working parents, and cultural biases which made these services unresponsive to the needs of inner-city residents. Neighborhood health centers were the proposed remedy: they would bring services to local communities and guarantee consumer participation through a system of advisory boards. A new group of paraprofessionals – physicians' assistants and nurse practitioners – promised to free physicians' time for important medical tasks and so offer improved and cheaper services to all consumers.

These strategies did not resolve the problem of access. Representatives on advisory boards did not have sufficient knowledge to counter the claims of medical experts, and did not genuinely represent the communities from which they were selected; the working poor still slipped through the cracks in the insurance system; paraprofessionals did not inspire enough confidence in the public and reimbursement for their services was set at the rate charged by the doctors who nominally supervised them. The failure of such measures raised doubts about the extent of consumer participation and the efficacy of a "voice strategy" in American health care.

The British NHS enjoyed great popularity after its inception in 1948. It certainly faced dilemmas in its first twenty years: how to cope with the changing health problems which came with a changing population structure? How to resolve competition and conflict among health care professionals over wages and differentials? How to improve administrative coordination among the various branches of the service – the hospital, the general practitioners, and the local authority health services – and how to improve the efficiency of the overall structure? To maximize the equitable distribution of resources, did one try to constrain the demands of the consumers of health care or of its producers (Klein 1983)? Yet, on the whole, the NHS was relatively free from criticism by the public. This may have been a cause or an effect of the lack of institutionalized representation of consumers in the service. Technically, they had even fewer avenues for exercising their voice than their American counterparts.

The weakness of participation became a matter of concern as the perceived problems of the two national health care systems changed. Access gave way to other issues in the 1960s and 1970s, not least because medicine itself was no longer immune to criticism. Even if public health measures and improved social conditions had been more effective in reducing mortality from infectious diseases than medical advances, in the public imagination this achievement was credited to medicine. How much more frustrating, then, that modern medical science appeared to be faltering in the struggle with its new adversaries, the chronic diseases. In this context, consumers were probably more unwilling to tolerate demeaning or unsatisfactory aspects of the medical relationship. For the sake of a fail-safe cure, they might overlook the absence of a reassuring bedside manner. Both popular culture and firsthand accounts of serious illness and the health care personnel who try to conquer it are full of images of cold, abrupt professionals who are nevertheless superb technicians, men and women who acquire flawed personal styles perhaps *because of* the fact that they are dedicated to science (see, for example, Lerner 1978: 74–5, 78–9, 97–9,

206–07; Lear 1980: 216–19, 235, 257–58, 389). But when medicine could promise neither relief nor cure, the quality of the relationship between patient and doctor assumed an even greater importance. Qualities of the *individual* physician were crucial when the efficacy of the profession as a whole was in question. The medical encounter could be searched for the clues which it might reveal about a physician's competence; it also constituted an important sphere of meaning in its own right.

Social movements in both countries attacked diverse aspects of the relationship between doctors and patients. Social critics like Ivan Illich, R.D. Laing, and Herbert Marcuse, whose work was read widely on both sides of the Atlantic, argued that citizens of western capitalist societies had lost a sense of their fundamental human potential and had delegated important social functions to a variety of experts. The task which now confronted them was to decode the language of expertise and to reclaim the essential human relationships at the heart of healing, education, work, and family life. The consumer movement indicted medicine because drugs and doctors had become downright dangerous in many instances, causing more damage than they cured. The women's movement's critique went deeper in that it questioned the nature of the relationship which existed between women and their doctors. Physicians controlled reproductive technology and had appropriated the traditional domestic knowledge of "old wives," mothers, and grandmothers; women should reclaim it. Moreover, by being party to the medical contract, women often had to concur in a world view that portrayed them first as "sickly," then as hysterical, and finally as neurotic or promiscuous, to obtain care (Ruzek 1979; Chamberlain 1981; Doyal 1983).

The critique of the social relationships inherent in medical institutions did not evolve separately from larger political and social developments. In both Britain and the United States, the "participation revolution" (Bell 1976) – the democratization of structures and the decline of attitudes supporting hierarchy – has been alternately lamented and celebrated. Samuel Beer (1982) describes the "collapse of deference" and the "romantic revolt" which characterized Britain in the 1960s and 1970s. The traditional bonds of social class and party, he argues, were weakened and undermined by a new antibureaucratic, participatory, and decentralizing ethos in both politics and culture. In the Unitd States, Daniel Bell chronicled the revolt against the idea of a meritocracy and the creation of "new social forms to involve people in crucial decisions" (Bell 1976: 203).

The demand for participation did not always incorporate an attack on the nature of the relationships which were intrinsic to hierarchical structures. The critiques of unyielding bureaucracies and of the mystification of the expert were probably carried furthest within social services and the professions. The American demand for "participatory democracy" gave rise to a range of alternative organizations which were to transform both living and working: free schools (Swidler 1979), law collectives, communes, free schools, and food co-ops (Case and Taylor 1979). Free clinics were designed not only to help underserved populations like minority communities, drug users, hippies, and victims of the new epidemic of venereal disease, but also to promulgate a new organizational model of service delivery. Their "prefigurative" purpose was to demonstrate in a restricted setting (they rarely aspired to provide services beyond good primary care) that an egalitarian, considerate, caring relationship was possible between practitioner and client. These organizations differed in many respects but they shared "a rejection of authority as a valid principle for regulating group life" (Swidler 1979: 2). They met with varying degrees of success. In education this social movement helped to transform the public school system. Free schools "failed" – that is, they disappeared – precisely because many of the innovations they fostered were adopted by conventional schools (Graubard 1979).

Medicine, on the other hand, resisted the new populist demands and the pressure for democratization. In the United States, free clinics either collapsed or continued to exist as a parallel system of primary care for the poor but their structural innovations and their efforts to change the relationship between health care personnel and clients were not adopted by conventional medical organizations. New planning organizations, Health System Agencies, failed to give consumers extensive control over the health care system and had no impact on the relationship between doctor and client. The women's movement has had some effect on the latter, but it has been restricted to specific aspects of the encounter between women and physicians, focusing on procedures such as pelvic examinations and abortions.

In Britain, the most recent effort to secure community involvement, Community Health Councils, were hailed as a "strong consumer voice both to criticize and champion the NHS" (Owen 1976, cited in USHP 1979: 56), but without adequate access to information or substantial formal powers they have remained comparatively weak. Moreover, their primary purpose was never to overhaul the existing dynamic of the doctor–patient relationship. Feminists in Britain have softened their attack on physicians and shifted the direction of their criticisms in recent years, dwelling less on the problems of medical sexism and more on the effects of cutbacks in the NHS on women and on women health workers (Doyal 1983).

The relationship between doctors and patients is, by and large, impervious to structural measures designed to enhance consumer participation, which, in any event, are usually oriented to give consumers a say in the *planning* or organization of health care services. Patients and their families are, indeed, buying a service when they come into contact with medical care, but – the more crucial component in calculations of satisfaction – they are also entering into a relationship. It is a relationship that possesses a number of peculiar features. Consumers, as many people have pointed out, do not necessarily know what they are getting from medical care. They cannot evaluate doctors the way they do blenders or automobiles. They do not always know if tests are required or what the appropriate length of a hospital stay is for one procedure versus another. They may not have the resources, time or energy to determine a particular specialist's record of cures and failures. What they do know, and what they can evaluate, is whether they like the way they are being treated and whether they instinctively feel that the man or woman across the desk is a "good doctor."

The criteria they employ in reaching this decision have been much debated by sociologists. Freidson (1961) found that doctors had to display both a quality of competence and an active interest in their patients for the latter to feel that they were receiving good medical care. Medical practice is a complex operation conducted at several different levels. At its heart is an authority relationship which depends for legitimation on the sanctioning of the profession's claims to knowledge and skill, but the frequent analogy made to the parent–child relationship (see the review by Wilson and Bloom 1972) indicates that it must also speak to patients' emotional needs. While the 1960s saw the beginning of a reworking of authority relationships in some spheres of social life – the family, the church, education – the relationship between practitioner and patient did not undergo any radical change in this period. It did not become more familial or egalitarian. Medicine shrugged off the demands of the 1960s. Instead, in the following decade, the changing political economy of medicine placed a new set of social pressures on physicians which, in turn, constrained the patient–practitioner relationship, making it more distant, less open and more conflictual.

The deterioration of the medical encounter

In the United States, the right to informed consent, won in the 1970s, constrains doctors to present fully the risks of treatment to patients, who can sue if they suffer harm after not being fully informed. Doctors, argues Kennedy, have become more cautious, "hiding behind consent forms . . . instead of talking to their patients" – the ironic effect of legal intervention that was intended to enhance dialogue between doctor and patient but that "has produced instead a monologue, in which the consent form is made to do the talking" (Kennedy 1983: 172). Malpractice suits have increased against doctors, who are more likely to practice defensively as a result. After 1970, the insurance industry, business and the state, alarmed for different reasons by the aggregate costs of health care, put increasing pressure on physicians, whom they saw as the critical decision makers (controlling amount of surgery and hospital care), and argued for more government regulation of the health care industry (Starr 1982).

In Britain, efforts in the 1970s to allocate health care funds and resources in an even fashion across the country and to eliminate private beds in the NHS challenged the monopoly of technical expertise in health-related decisions. Physicians felt beleaguered. The 1974 reorganization of the NHS simply produced a greater structural complexity which drew complaints from those working within it.

Such constraints exacerbated long-run trends which were reshaping the medical encounter in ways that proved increasingly onerous to patients. With the growth of specialization, most notably in the United States, the opportunity for a continuous, close relationship with a doctor who knows a patient and his or her family well has declined; communication of information about illness on the part of both patient and doctor is impeded by a variety of structural and cultural factors (Waitzkin and Stoeckle 1976); the locus of decision making in the hospital setting appears ever more remote. Technological interventions and "breakthroughs" in chronic illnesses, such as heart disease and kidney failure, can prolong life sometimes at the cost of its quality. Clinical staff, faced with new disease entities (end stage renal disease replaces protracted death), have to cope with a range of untidy, unmanageable problems created by the "biological and social complexity" which the patient represents. The temptations to take refuge in a clinical construction of illness which denies the patient's experience are enormous (Plough 1981). The general mystification of medical procedures and knowledge is exacerbated for technological reasons and, because situations of medical uncertainty are hard for doctors and patients alike, for psychological reasons. Finally, pushing dissatisfaction with what a doctor does or how he or she acts to the level of open conflict is always difficult.

A review of the procedures for dealing with consumer complaints in the NHS ten years ago argued that there were numerous obstacles to instituting satisfactory outlets for consumer dissatisfaction which were

> inherent in the organization and attitudes of the health professions, especially the doctors, and in the structure of the service itself. . . . First, the socio-cultural differences between many consumers and the providers of the service; second, the hierarchical structure of the National Health Service; third, the newly-invented divorce between 'management' and 'consumer'; and fourth, the claims of certain professionals, especially the doctors, to "clinical autonomy."   (Stacey 1973: 11)

With a little modification, this statement still applies. The Health Service Commissioner, created in 1974 to deal with patient complaints, was not permitted to deal with cases which involved questions of clinical autonomy (Klein 1983).

For all these reasons, consumers have found it hard to work out what a "voice option" would be with regard to the medical encounter (how does one articulate grievances and act to change a relationship with one's physician?), let alone how they might exercise it. But an "exit option" is also increasingly denied them. In Britain, leaving the NHS is not a viable choice for any but the middle class who can afford private health insurance. Despite alarmist noises by the recent Thatcher administration, the private sector in health care is still very small. Changing doctors within the NHS is viewed as very difficult by patients (Stimson and Webb 1975); the administrative procedures for arranging through a Family Practitioner Committee to transfer to another general practitioner (who controls access to hospital care and to specialists) are cumbersome and often entail delays just when patients feel that they can least afford them.

In the United States, changing doctors is theoretically easier, but in practice it is a time-consuming and potentially emotionally exhausting task. Group insurance plans are usually offered as part of a benefit package at work: transferring from one of the two or three plans that an employer may offer to another is often permitted only once a year, with extended waiting periods before coverage under the new plan commences. Not all plans will cover "second opinions," seeking advice from a second doctor as to whether a procedure is really necessary. With new group practice arrangements or Health Maintenance Organizations (HMOs), patients are fearful that their objections to certain kinds of treatment by a doctor or other health care personnel may follow them in the form of a reputation for being "difficult" patients, since one does not quit the organization when one quits a particular physician.

Within the confines of conventional medicine, patients are forced, therefore, to confront the many problematic aspects of the relationship with a physician which are peculiar to modern medical practice, and find no easy mechanism at hand to change it. Simultaneously, the larger social context of medicine structures their perceptions and experience in new ways so that the demands they make of doctors and health care change, as do their reservations about the medical encounter.

First, at the most immediate level, is the question of whether patients feel that they are being treated with respect. Confidence on this score seems to be down. The social context of interaction has become more charged since the consumer movement, the civil rights movement, and the women's movement have brought the issue of sexist or racist attitudes on the part of health care personnel into public consciousness. In Britain, complaints about the health care system often center on the problem of queues: crowded waiting rooms and long waits for elective surgical procedures engender charges that patients are being treated like ciphers. In the United States, new legal and social pressures threaten to erode the treasured principle of doctor–patient confidentiality. When members of group practice teams, nonmedical employees in hospitals and insurance personnel may see an individual's medical record, or part of it, and when laws require physicians and other health care personnel to report perpetrators of child molestation, and patients suffering from bullet wounds, or certain kinds of sexually transmitted diseases, confidentiality is easily breached (Cleere 1967; Altman 1983; *New York Times* 1984).

Second, in the context of a much touted "information revolution," medical knowledge has become a burgeoning industry. Consumers from every social class are bombarded with "medical facts" from popular magazines (Taylor and Mattes 1980), from self-help books and from television programs which range from consulting the doctor on the air to the NOVA documentary. When the "educated consumer" can read up on the details of his or her illness or symptoms, it might be expected that middle-class patients in particular will become frustrated by the continuing defense on the part of the medical profession of the principle of clinical autonomy. State regulation of the profession may have increased, but it does not extend to challenging the principle that only physicians are in the position to review, let alone challenge, the clinical judgments of other physicians.

Third, as Rosenberg (1979) has argued in the case of the physician in the middle of the nineteenth century, doctors have to create therapeutic regimens which are emotionally as well as intellectually meaningful. And, although patients and doctors are no longer united by the same view of the body and the determinants of disease, the efficacy of the physician is still frequently measured against the yardstick of whether he or she is "doing something." The capacity of the doctor to meet this criterion has been undermined in several ways. With changing disease patterns, the number of patients who live with chronic pain has increased. In many instances, the treatment of choice is to do nothing, to advocate rest and inaction and to entrust decisions about extent of movement to the *patient's* better judgment. Such recommendations may increase a patient's sense of control but they may also prove frustrating and frightening and, most important, they leave the doctor in a position where, symbolically, he or she has nothing to offer and nothing to do. Most classes of modern drugs, with a few exceptions, produce no dramatic physiological effect on the patient who takes them (Rosenberg 1979: 21); the patient has to rely on the doctor's word that something is being done.

Finally, cultural images of patients and consumers of medical services are changing. As consumers enter into a contract with the health care system and a relationship with a physician, they are subscribing to or reinforcing an imagery about themselves and their complaints which is embodied in that relationship. In the early 1980s this entails submitting to a set of moral judgments about their behavior which are both negative and contradictory. Many observers have remarked on the popularity within health policy circles of theories about the sources of modern illness that place most of the responsibility for it on the shoulders of consumers and patients (Crawford 1979; Taylor 1982). Personal self-destructive habits – smoking, drinking alcohol to excess, lack of exercise, eating too much and badly – rather than social, occupational, and environmental conditions are believed to be the "risk factors" that predispose people to contract cancer, heart disease, and stroke (Breslow 1980). Yet neither the state nor the medical profession has relinquished control over the management of health care and the organization of services. Along with the rhetoric about people shouldering responsibility for the medical problems they have brought upon themselves goes another rhetoric: that consumers by and large cannot be trusted to make appropriate decisions about their health care – they shop around for services in a disorganized inept fashion, they use too many services and enter the health care system at the wrong point.

Recent American solutions to the latter problem have been

couched in terms of an appeal to the power of the market. New incentives are needed to make consumers into more prudent buyers of medical services and to induce competition into health care markets. The HMO strategy is being revamped to achieve both ends (Brown 1981). The British solution consists in more efficient organization and more rigorous state intervention. Despite Margaret Thatcher's nods in the direction of the private sector, the major strategy to contain health care costs and to dissuade consumers from careless and self-indulgent action has been to try to cap the spending of local health authorities. In some areas these measures, together with manpower cuts, have constrained the flow of patients among services and regions (Glick and Offen 1983). Both the American and the British strategies have imposed further pressures on both physicians and patients, which can do little to build a relaxed and trusting relationship between them. They have also reinforced a new cultural ideal about how patients ought to behave and a set of moral judgments about how they are falling short of that ideal. Consumers are simultaneously exhorted to be more responsible about their habits and told that they cannot be trusted to be responsible about their use of services so that their health care must be "managed" for them.

These developments suggest that it is not public disenchantment with science that has led to a disillusionment with medicine, but a fall in public regard for *doctors*. The proportion of the population having "a great deal of confidence" in medicine fell in the United States from 73 per cent in 1966 to 42 per cent in 1976 (Harris poll cited in Starr 1978: 178). In contrast to Paul Starr (1982: 393), who has argued that Americans are more hostile to doctors as a class while they retain confidence in their own personal physicians, I suspect that people's individual negative experiences with doctors have undermined their optimism about the profession. Recent British surveys find that "nearly a quarter of the United Kindom population say that they have less faith in doctors than they used to; and the number of those who 'trust the doctor to know what I need' fell from 52 per cent in 1978 to 39 per cent in 1980" (West and Inglis 1983a: 6).

The rigidities of and flaws in the medical encounter might not have been experienced as so irksome except for the fact that, as the personal relationship between practitioner and patient became more attenuated, both the institution of medicine and the question of health were becoming more central in people's lives. Sontag (1978) may not have been accurate in all respects in her provocative account of how the current imagery about cancer reflects contemporary fears about the direction of modern society, but *Illness as Metaphor* provided an important confirmation of the degree to which Americans have become obsessed with their health. The current interest in fitness may reflect the popularization of new scientific findings about the hidden dangers of a sedentary lifestyle and a driven Type A personality, but more likely it crystallizes concerns that are inspired by broader social changes.

Medicine has acquired enormous political and cultural significance as its jurisdiction over social life has been extended. Birth and death have been defined as medical events. Problems which used to be the sole responsibility of the church or the courts – juvenile delinquency, divorce, crimes of passion – now fall in great part to medicine for resolution. Doctors are the gatekeepers to many benefits such as sickness compensation and abortion, and major protagonists in a host of complicated social decisions required to resolve controversies about who has the right to die, who is dangerous to themselves and their community, who may conceive children and who can obtain a new lease on life through an organ transplant. Visions of unlimited technical advances in medical care are now tempered by concerns about the growing "medicalization" of social life and personal troubles. Paradoxically, the sense of entitlement which the 1960s are supposed to have brought about, particularly with regard to consumers and their services, has probably led to a situation where patients want and expect *more* from their doctors just as, for different reasons, both the managers of services and social critics are instructing them to ask for less.

Exit to a new relationship?

Some part of the resurgence of alternative medicines, therefore, can be explained by popular dissatisfaction with medicine. But it is not the fact that modern science cannot always cure them that provides consumers with the impetus to try something different, but the fact that the fragile and complex relationship between healer and healed is collapsing, placed under enormous pressure at a time when the bases of authority relationships in many other social institutions have changed, when health has become a popular obsession (especially in America), and when the institution of medicine has become more central than ever before in people's lives. In such circumstances, given the general intractability of the health care system, new social pressures which have produced intransigence on the part of the medical profession, and almost universal uncertainty as to how one might rework the medical encounter, exit becomes a rational choice. As the number of alternative practitioners rises, as many of the legal restrictions on them are removed and as insurance provisions cover an increasing number of alternative therapies, it also becomes a plausible choice.

Exit is not for everyone all the time, of course. What consumers, who have rejected the conventional medical relationship, then decide to do will depend to some degree on what options are available to them. They are likely to endure an unsatisfactory relationship when faced with a life-threatening condition that modern medicine can cure. They are more likely to embark on a search for a relationship more to their taste when the financial costs are not prohibitive. What they do will also depend on the kind of relationship they do or do not want. Patients vary in the degree to which they want information, in their reactions to being given more control over treatment strategies, and in their preferences for more or less direction from physicians (Krantz, Baum, and Wideman 1980). Preferences also vary by race, class, and gender as well as by individual temperament and psychology.

Nevertheless, I suspect that systematic investigation would reveal that trends in the popularity of different alternative medicines in both Britain and the United States could be illuminated by asking, first, what are the constraints on doctors and patients that jeopardize their relationship in different ways and, second, in contrast, what kind of relationship between practitioner and patient do various alternative healing systems offer? For the moment, such an argument must remain speculative since very few studies exist which actually ask patients why they consult alternative practitioners. Looking at what we know about the characteristics of alternative therapies, however, provides some basis to argue that it is the nature of the encounter between practitioner and patient which may help to explain the similarities and differences in the clientele for alternative medicines in two western nations.

Homoeopathy, for example, is a system of healing in which the patient is expected to accept the authority of the trained expert – "in the hands of *a skilled practitioner. . . .*homoeopathy can cure anything that's curable" (cited in Romano 1980: 31, emphasis mine) – but which promises a relationship with a healer who will spend a great deal of time with each client and design a course of treatment tailored to his or her particular temperament, history, and peculiarities. The medical correspondent of a British newspaper, asked to evaluate homoeopathy, concluded that

> perhaps the most striking feature . . . was "the doctor's attitude towards the patient." As in orthodox medicine, the first step with a new patient is history-taking, "but history-taking with a difference. Not only are the diagnostic symptoms considered, but also the patient's personality and constitution – physiological and psychological – as manifested in temperament and disposition." Even his or her likes and dislikes are taken into consideration.
>
> (Inglis and West 1983: 70)

The emphasis, then, is on the individual and not the disease or the "case." "Homeopathy," argues Stanway, "is 'whole person' medicine" in that it takes into account "domestic, personal and psychological as well as frankly medical aspects of the illness" (Stanway 1982: 159). Not only does it consider the person's total environment but it enlists the help of the patient's network of relatives and friends to diagnose illness:

> The patient's family can be of considerable assistance to the doctor who may not know that patient's mannerisms so well and thus not spot so easily any divergence from normal. Many a homeopathic remedy has been successfully prescribed as a result of a member of a patient's family remarking on some small trait in the patient which has only appeared during the course of the illness.
>
> (Ainsworth 1979: 116)

Whereas homoeopathy offers intensive personal attention and

an individualized program of treatment, from a qualified expert who is often (especially in Britain) also trained as a conventional physician, acupuncture frequently demands more active participation from the patient. Particularly with regard to the treatment of addictive disorders,

> Acupuncturists who practice holistically like to make it clear from the start that theirs is not a form of treatment which depends simply on correct diagnosis and accurate positioning of needles during treatment, with the patient as passive onlooker while everything is done to and for him or her. On the contrary, all that acupuncture can do for many disorders is, in effect, to tune up the system; they emphasize the patient must do the rest.   (Inglis and West 1983: 124)

For those patients who elect acupuncture because of its efficacy as an analgesic, surgery becomes a much less mysterious process because they are active observers, awake and aware throughout the various stages of treatment.

In both acupuncture and chiropractic, patient and practitioner are bound together by participating in an experience where there is tangible intervention on the part of the healer – manipulation of the spine or insertion of needles – an almost aggressive laying-on-of-hands. Although healer and patient may not share the same body metaphors, although the patient may not understand or, indeed, care about the epistemological basis of the physician's science, nevertheless, he or she can see and often feel (unlike the experience of the homoeopathic patient) that something is being done. The clientele of spiritual healers may prefer a relationship with a charismatic individual in which the authority of the healer is vested in personal qualities rather than demonstrable therapeutic skills. The members of self-help groups, in contrast, do not seek to reshape the personal relationship with a medical expert but, instead, take comfort in a relationship with a collectivity. Shared experience is the central component in the strategy of groups modeled on Alcoholics Anonymous and self-help programs for the victims of a wide range of afflictions: drug addicts, cancer patients, and the parents of children with Down's Syndrome (Withorn 1980).

The increasing trend towards "self-care" (individual lay measures to prevent and to treat health problems, such as monitoring symptoms, administering medications and even engaging in fairly complicated medical interventions) in both countries (Helman 1981; Rosenzweig 1978) seems, at first glance, to be the exception to this argument because it represents not a search for a new relationship with healers but rather a rejection of any relationship at all. It has been described as the extreme manifestion of a popular desire to "reduce doctor-dependence" (Yeager 1977: 44). At the same time it accepts the premises and paraphernalia of modern medical practice. A welter of self-care manuals, training programs, and courses now exist to teach patients to "assume more responsibility for their own health" by doing much of what they have previously entrusted to doctors. Mothers learn how to take throat cultures and diagnose ear infections, astronauts are taught how to immobilize broken bones, women can take Pap smears, and anyone can learn to use stethoscopes and blood pressure cuffs (Yeager 1977: 43). It may be, therefore, that for some patients going to the doctor has become such an unpleasant experience that they are anxious to avoid the medical encounter altogether. They can do this for a host of minor ailments. They may also be the patients who, while they believe in medical science, want more control over their health.

The medical profession for its part, one might assume, should be alarmed that playing doctor, which used to be a game for kids, is now a serious adult preoccupation. Andrews and Levin (1979), for example, predict that do-it-yourself health texts or health education programs may be attacked under existing medical practice acts because they pose an "economic threat to organized medicine" (p. 47), even greater than the isolated actions of individuals who use some version of self-medication. Physicians, however, seem to have embraced self-care wholeheartedly for the simple reason that they see it as a complement rather than a challenge to their own activities and no threat to professional jurisdiction or privilege. If patients were to practice self-care, unnecessary visits to the doctor's office could be avoided (Yeager 1977; Gartner 1982), "medically savvy" patients would be more inclined to follow their doctor's advice, the overall costs of health care would be reduced (Gartner 1982) and physicians would not be held accountable for every aspect of medical treatment and so blamed unjustly for everything that goes wrong (Staver 1977).

Experiments in which high school graduates were trained how to use computer-based protocols to care for patients with a variety of diseases, demonstrated that self-care could achieve a 20 per cent saving in physician time (Yeager 1977).

A movement which promises to deliver a new generation of compliant, intelligent patients and to provide relief from both onerous responsibilities and trivial medical tasks obviously holds many attractions for a beleaguered profession. More important, it does not undermine professional authority since it neither denies the efficacy of modern medicine nor criticizes its practitioners. It is a movement which sees doctor and patient working in harmony. Most of the time its adherents assume the role of apprentices and look for direction to medically trained personnel who insist, by and large, that "any self-care program should be carefully co-ordinated under the supervision of one's own physician" (Yeager 1977: 49). The patient can avoid medical encounters or reduce their number and the doctor, although invisible, can remain in control.

Conclusion

Viewing the renewed interest in alternative medicines in this way highlights the similarities in their development in Britain and the United States. It minimizes the role of cultural differences between the two countries, and of other factors to which the emergence of alternative systems of healing have been attributed. The tenuousness of orthodox medicine's "legitimacy" in the United States (Wallis and Morley 1976: 17), the fact that the practice of alternative forms of therapy is a customary right in Britain (Fulder and Monro 1981: 4), the monopoly of service by the NHS – "once limited by state control medical enterprise has not been free to respond to patient demand and has been fettered by government finance" (Rogers 1983) – I argue, are of much less importance in explaining the resurgence of alternative medicines than the changing quality of the medical encounter. The relationship between doctor and patient has been altered in a somewhat different fashion in Britain and America, but in both countries it has been subjected to enormous constraints and to criticism from laymen and professionals alike.

Focusing on the relationship between doctor and patient also restores a neglected dimension to the histories of medicine on both sides of the Atlantic. Most of the latter have concentrated on the development and organization of the medical profession; the patient remains invisible or, perhaps worse, exists as a static universal figure, whose demands and perceptions do not change over time and are not informed by emerging cultural movements or economic developments. Medicine, however, as I have insisted throughout this paper, is a relationship; its growth and its failings cannot be understood without taking into account the dynamic interaction between patient and physician, viewed as a historical phenomenon.

The eventual fate of alternative healing systems is, of course, contingent on many structural and organizational factors of the kind that Wardwell (1976) has explored with regard to the likely trajectory of chiropractic: How much opposition do they engender from the medical profession? Will the state accord them legal recognition? What is the degree of solidarity or fragmentation within the alternative practitioner group? But if, as I have argued, one of the critical reasons for the public's disillusionment with conventional medicine is their frustration over the kind of relationship which obtains between doctor and patient, coupled with a perception that their circumstances permit them either to avoid it outright or to continue the search for something different and better, then among the most important factors to consider in assessing the future of alternative medicines in both Britain and the United States will be those that affect the nature of the medical encounter.

Note

1 Throughout this paper I have used the terms healing and healers in their colloquial sense to mean a system and its practitioners which claim to restore a sick person to a state of health. When I refer to the body of men and women who believe in the existence of a healing force, either divine or natural, which can be tapped by them and so channeled through them to the sick, I use the terms spiritual healing and spiritual healer.

References

Africano, L. (1975) Acupuncture: Child of the Media. *The Nation* 220: 657–60.

Ainsworth, J.B.L. (1979) Homeopathy. In M. Hulke (ed.) *The Encyclopedia of Alternative Medicine and Self-Help*. New York: Schocken Books.

Altman, L.K. (1983) Physician–Patient Confidentiality Slips Away. *The New York Times* (27 September): Cl.

Andrews, L.B. and Levin, L.S. (1979) Self-Care and the Law. *Social Policy* 9: 44–9.

Atkinson, P. (1978) From Honey to Vinegar: Levi- Strauss in Vermont. In P. Morley and R. Wallis (eds) *Culture and Curing: Anthropological Perspectives on Traditional Medical Beliefs and Practices*. London: Peter Owen.

Avina, R.L. and Schneiderman, L.J. (1978) Why Patients Choose Homeopathy (commentary). *The Western Journal of Medicine* 128 (4): 366–9.

Beer, S.H. (1982) *Britain Against Itself: The Political Contradictions of Collectivism*. New York: W.W. Norton.

Bell, D. (1976) *The Cultural Contradictions of Capitalism*. New York: Basic Books.

Berliner, H. (1982) Medical Modes of Production. In P. Wright and A. Treacher (eds) *The Problem of Medical Knowledge*. New York: Columbia University Press.

Berliner, H.S. and Salmon, J.W. (1980) The Holistic Alternative to Scientific Medicine: History and Analysis. *International Journal of Health Services* 10(1): 133–47.

Breslow, L. (1980) Risk Factor Intervention for Health Maintenance. In D. Mechanic (ed.) *Readings in Medical Sociology*. New York: The Free Press.

Brown, L.D. (1981) Competition and Health Cost Containment: Cautions and Conjectures. *Milbank Memorial Fund Quarterly, Health and Society* 59(2): 145–89.

Brown, R.E. (1979) *Rockefeller Medicine Men: Medicine and Capitalism in America*. Berkeley: University of California Press.

Callan, J.P. (1979) Holistic Health or Holistic Hoax? (editorial). *JAMA* 241(11): 1156.

Case, J. and Taylor, R.C.R. (eds) (1979) *Co-ops, Communes and Collectives*. New York: Pantheon Books.

Chamberlain, M. (1981) *Old Wives' Tales: Their History, Remedies and Spells*. London: Virago Press.

Cleary, P.D. (1982) Chiropractic Use: A Test of Several Hypotheses. *American Journal of Public Health* 72 (7): 727–30.

Cleere, R.L., Dougherty, W.J., Fiumara, N.J., Jenike, C., Leutz, J.W., and Rose, N.J (1967) Physicians' Attitudes Toward Venereal Disease Reporting. *Journal of the American Medical Association* 202 (10): 921–46.

Crawford, R. (1979) Individual Responsibility and Health Politics in the 1970s. In S. Reverby and D. Rosner (eds) *Health Care in America*. Philadelphia: Temple University Press.

Culliton, B.J. and Waterfall, W.K. (1979) Chiropractors and the AMA. *The British Medical Journal* 1: 467–68.

Doyal, L. (1983) Women, Health and the Sexual Division of Labour: A Case Study of the Women's Health Movement in Britain. *Critical Social Policy* 3(1): 21–33.

Dunea, G. (1979) Healing by Touching. *British Medical Journal* 1: 795–96.

Eagle, R. (1978) On the Fringe. *Observer Magazine* (21 May): 31–47.

——(1980) *A Guide to Alternative Medicine*. London: The British Broadcasting Corporation.

Firman, G.J. and Goldstein, M.S. (1975) The Future of Chiropractic: A Psychosocial View. *The New England Journal of Medicine* 293(13): 639–42.

Freidson, E. (1961) *Patient Views of Medical Practice*. New York: Russell Sage Foundation.

Fulder, S. and Monro, R. (1981) *The Status of Complementary Medicine in the United Kingdom*. London: The Threshold Foundation Bureau.

Gartner, A. (1982) Self-Help/Self-Care: A Cost-Effective Health Strategy. *Social Policy* 12 (4): 64.

Glick, I.W. and Offen D.N. (1983) Letter. *The Times* (10 August): 9.

Graubard, A. (1979) From Free Schools to "Educational Alternatives". In J. Case and R.C.R. Taylor (eds) *Co-ops, Communes and Collectives*. New York: Pantheon Books.

Halberstam, M. (1976) Holistic Healing: Limits of "The New Medicine." *Psychology Today* 9: 24–5.

Harrell, D.E. (1975) *All Things are Possible*. Bloomington: Indiana University Press.

Hassett, J. (1980) Acupuncture is Proving its Points. *Psychology Today* 14 (12): 81–82ff.

Helman, C. (1981) Feed a Cold, Starve a Fever. *New Society* (5 November): 223–5.

Hirschman, A.O. (1970) *Exit, Voice, and Loyalty: Responses to Decline in Firms, Organizations, and States*. Cambridge, Mass.: Harvard University Press.

Holden, C. (1978) Holistic Health Concepts Gaining Momentum. *Science* 200: 1029.

Hulke, M. (ed.) (1979) *The Encyclopedia of Alternative Medicine and Self-Help*. New York: Schocken Books.

Illich, I. (1977) *Medical Nemesis: The Expropriation of Health*. New York: Bantam Books.

Inglis, B. and West, R. (1983) *The Alternative Health Guide*. London: Michael Joseph.

Kane, R.L. *et al.* (1974) Manipulating the Patient: a Comparison of the Effectiveness of Physician and Chiropractor Care. *Lancet* 1: 1333–336.

Kennedy, I. (1983) *The Unmasking of Medicine*. London: Paladin Books, Granada.

Klein, R. (1983) *The Politics of the National Health Service*. New York: Longman Inc.

Krantz, D.S., Baum, A., and Wideman, M. (1980) Assessment of Preferences for Self-Treatment and Information in Health Care. *Journal of Personality and Social Psychology* 39(5): 977–90.

Lear, M.W. (1980) *Heartsounds: The Story of a Love and Loss*. New York: Simon & Shuster.

Lee, J.A. (1976) Social Change and Marginal Therapeutic Systems. In R. Wallis and P. Morley (eds) *Marginal Medicine*. London: Peter Owen.

Lerner, G. (1978) *A Death of One's Own*. New York: Harper & Row.

New York Times (1984) California Child Held in Contempt. (8 January): 19.

Owen, D. (1976) *In Sickness and Health*. London: Quartet.

Parker, G. and Tupling, H. (1977) Consumer Evaluation of Natural Therapists and General Practitioners. *The Medical Journal of Australia* 1: 619–22.

Parliamentary Correspondent (1978) Homeopathic Medicine. *The Lancet* 2(8081): 166–67.

Parssinen, T.M. (1979) Professional Deviants and the History of Medicine: Medical Mesmerists in Victorian Britain. In R. Wallis (ed.) *On the Margins of Science: The Social Construction of Rejected Knowledge*. University of Keele, Keele, Staffordshire: Sociological Review Monograph 27.

Plough, A.L. (1981) Medical Technology and the Crisis of Experience: The Costs of Clinical Legitimation. *Social Science and Medicine* 15F: 89–101.

Roebuck, J. and Quan, R. (1976) Health-Care Practices in the American Deep South. In R. Wallis and P. Morley (eds) *Marginal Medicine*. London: Peter Owen.

Rogers, A.R. (1983) Letter. *The Times* (16 August): 11.

Romano, D.L. (1980) The Return of Homeopathy. *Ms* 9: 30–7 + .

Rosenberg, C.E. (1979) The Therapeutic Revolution. In M.J. Vogel and C.E. Rosenberg (eds) *The Therapeutic Revolution*. Philadelphia: University of Pennsylvania Press.

Rosenzweig, S. (1978) Learning To Be Your Own MD. *New York*

Times Magazine (2 April): 42–6.

Rossman, M. (1975) The Orthodox and Unorthodox in Health Care. *Social Policy* 6: 28–30.

Rubin, L.S. (1979) Biofeedback: Medicine's Newest Cure-All? *Family Health* 11: 50–3 + .

Ruzek, S.B. (1979) *The Women's Health Movement*. New York: Praeger Publishers.

Rynearson, E.H. (1974) Americans Love Hogwash. *Nutrition Reviews* 32 (supplement): 1–14.

Salmon, J.W. and Berliner, H.S. (1980a) Health Policy Implications of the Holistic Health Movement. *Journal of Health Politics, Policy and Law* 5(3): 535–53.

Salmon, J.W. and Berliner, H.S. (1980b) The Holistic Health Movement: Challenges to Health Care and Health Planning. *American Journal of Acupuncture* 8(3): 197–203.

Sechrist, W.C (1979) Total Wellness and Holistic Health: A Bandwagon We Cannot Afford to Jump Onto! *Health Education* (September/October): 27.

Sontag, S. (1978) *Illness as Metaphor*. New York: Random House.

Stacey, M. (1973) Consumer Complaints Procedures in the British National Health Service. The Wade Marshall Memorial Lecture, presented at the annual meeting of the Society for the Study of Social Problems (August), New York.

Stanway, A. (1982) *Alternative Medicine*. New York: Penguin Books.

Starr, P. (1978) Medicine and the Waning of Professional Sovereignty. *Daedalus* (winter): 175–93.

——(1982) *The Social Transformation of American Medicine*. New York: Basic Books.

Staver, S. (1977) Self-Care Movement Gains Steam. *American Medical News* 20 (5 December): 14–15.

Stimson, G. and Webb, B. (1975) *Going to See the Doctor: The Consultation Process in General Practice*. London and Boston: Routledge & Kegan Paul.

Swidler, A. (1979) *Organization Without Authority: Dilemmas of Social Control in Free Schools*. Cambridge: Harvard University Press.

Taylor, R.C.R. (Summer 1982) The Politics of Prevention. *Social Policy* 13(1): 32–61.

Taylor, R.C.R. and Mattes, S. (1980) Women's Health and Women's Magazines. Paper presented at the 108th meeting of the American Public Health Association (19–23 October), Detroit, Michigan.

Twemlow, S.W. and Chamberlin, C.R. (1981) Holistic Medicine: Rethinking Attitudes Towards Health Care. *The Journal of the Kansas Medical Society* 82(10): 447–50 + .

Unit for the Study of Health Policy (USHP) (1979) *Rethinking*

Community Medicine: Towards a Renaissance in Public Health?
London: USHP.

Waitzkin, H. and Stoeckle, J.D. (1976) Information and Control and the Micro-Politics of Health Care. *Social Science and Medicine* 6 (June): 263–76.

Wallis, R. and Morley, P. (1976) Introduction. In R. Wallis and P. Morley (eds) *Marginal Medicine*. London: Peter Owen.

Walton, S. (1979) Holistic Medicine. *Science News* 116: 410–12.

Wardwell, W.I. (1976) Orthodox and Unorthodox Practitioners: Changing Relationships and the Future Status of Chiropractors. In R. Wallis and P. Morley (eds) *Marginal Medicine*. London: Peter Owen.

Wardwell, W. (1980) Sounding Board: The Future of Chiropractic. *New England Journal of Medicine* 302(12): 688–90.

West, R. and Inglis, B. (1983a) If the Mind is Fit, the Body Will Cure Itself. *The Times* (8 August): 6.

West, R. and Inglis, B. (1983b) New Path to the Roots of Illness. *The Times* (9 August): 6.

West, R. and Inglis, B. (1983c) Time to Shake the Medicine. *The Times* (10 August): 6.

White, M. and Skipper, J.F. (1971) The Chiropractic Physician: A Study of Career Contingencies. *Journal of Health and Social Behavior* 12: 300–06.

Williams, G. III. (1976) Biofeedback: Easing the Pain of Headache. *Science Digest* 79: 76–81.

Wilson, R.N. and Bloom, S.W. (1972) Patient-Practitioner Relationships. In H. Freeman, S. Levine, and L. Reeder (eds) *Handbook of Medical Sociology*. Englewood Cliffs, New Jersey: Prentice-Hall.

Withorn, A. (1980) Helping Ourselves: The Limits and Potential of Self Help. *Social Policy* (November/December): 25–39.

Yeager, R.C. (1977) The Self-Care Surge. *Medical World News* 18 (3 October): 43 + .

Yesalis, C.E., Wallace, R.B., Fisher, W.P., and Tokheim, R. (1980) Does Chiropractic Utilization Substitute for Less Available Medical Services? *American Journal of Public Health* 70(4): 415–17.

Acknowledgement

I am grateful for conversations with Peter Hall, whose suggestions and criticisms strengthened the argument of this paper, and for the comments of Jack Salmon, editor of this volume.

Eight

Holistic health centers
in the United States

James S. Gordon

During the last fifteen years, a broad-based challenge has arisen
to the prevailing biomedical model of health care, to the services which it dictates, the institutions in which these services
are delivered, and the research and training which sustain it.
Professionals concerned with public health and preventive
medicine have deepened their critique of the economic, industrial, social, environmental, and institutional conditions
which endanger health and frustrate effective health care.
While prominent writers, among them Leon Eisenberg (1977)
and George Engel (1977) have issued a call for a systems-based
"biopsychosocial" approach to health and illness, holistic physicians, and countless other providers and consumers have
begun to create a new kind of health care practice (Gordon
1980).

The structure of this holistic approach is informed by the
experience of the free clinic movement of the 1960s with its
emphasis on easy access, respectful treatment, patient
education, and self-care. Its tone owes much to the human
potential movement with its attention to individual

expressivity, personal growth in illness as well as in health, and the mutuality of the therapeutic encounter. Its practice is based on heightened respect for the uniqueness of each patient, an attention to the familial and social factors affecting health and illness, a faith in the individual's capacity for self-help and self-healing, and an amalgam of alternative and conventional, ancient and modern therapeutic techniques (Gordon 1978).

Although this approach to health care has been adopted by individual practitioners within and outside of the medical establishment, it has been most fully elaborated within the context of multi-disciplinary therapeutic and educational holistic health centers. After a brief discussion of the concepts of holism in health care and the historical origins of holistic health centers, I will outline some of the most salient characteristics of these centers. Finally, I will discuss the implications of this new institutional form for the practice of medicine and the future of health care.

Holism and holistic health

The concept of holism, and the word itself, was first introduced by the South African statesman and philosopher Jan Christian Smuts in his 1926 book, *Holism and Evolution*. To Smuts, holism (derived from the Greek "holos" or "holo", meaning whole) was a way of comprehending and describing whole organisms and systems as entities greater than and different from the sum of their parts, an antidote to the analytic reductionism of the prevailing sciences.

In the last several years, the adjective holistic – and its Anglicized cousin "wholistic" – has been revived and applied and misapplied to almost every human endeavor from jogging to home building. This is not surprising. The feeling that our society and its functions are becoming increasingly fragmented and specialized is widespread. At a time when narrow perspectives and single solutions appear inadequate to our problems, holism has emerged as a potential antidote, a catchall for our hopes.

The practice of medicine, that curious hybrid of art and science that affects all our lives so intimately, has been particularly influenced by technology and its imperatives toward specialization. In recent years, it has become the most fertile ground for the elaboration of a holistic perspective and practice.

It has become clear that the kinds of technology that helped to cure or correct infectious diseases are of little avail in coping with environmentally influenced, stress related, and "mental" illnesses, hypertension, diabetes, cancer, depression, alcoholism, insomnia which now account for the vast majority of our morbidity and mortality. We have become painfully aware of the biological, economic, and interpersonal side effects of an overmedicated and fragmented system of health care. In the wake of the Civil Rights, anti-war, and women's movements, increasing numbers of consumers – and professionals – have become willing to question and challenge this system to create alternatives which redress some of its excesses while maintaining the very real gains biomedicine has made (Gordon 1981).

Holistic medicine is the rubric under which many of these diverse alternatives are placed. Though it sometimes falls into the same trap as the orthodox system it criticizes – an excessive and faddish reliance on particular techniques, a dogmatic rejection of its critics – it does postulate a longer and different view of health care. It respects the patients' capacity for healing themselves and regards them as active partners in health care rather than passive recipients. It does not neglect the occasional need for swift and authoritative medical or surgical intervention, but does put them in a context of care which emphasizes health promotion and patient education, and a reliance on modalities which patients themselves can implement – nutrition, exercise, relaxation techniques, and changes in attitude.

Though it is sometimes contrasted with them, the holistic approach to medicine includes "humanistic medicine" (which reflects a particular *attitude* toward health care, emphasizes the relationship between physicians and patients, and the psychological and spiritual development of both the patient and the physician), "psychosomatic medicine" (which reflects an enlarged *perspective* on illness and is concerned with the interdependence and mutual influence of psychological and physical factors), and "behavioral medicine" (which broadens the psychosomatic perspective to include the psychosocial causes and effects of illness). Though no one practice actually does so, holistic medicine does attempt to enlarge the continuum of health care. Ideally it includes the humanistic attitudes and the psychosomatic, behavioral and public health perspectives as well as any of the techniques which modern science and empirical use have revealed to be helpful: biofeedback and meditation, psychotherapy and behavior modification, modern fluid replacement and ancient acupuncture, diet and drugs, surgery and massage.

Holistic health is a broader if less precise concept. On the one hand, it means a state in which body, mind, and spirit are functioning in an integrated way in a supportive environment. On the other, it denotes a largely unorganized group of holistic physicians and nonphysicians, of health care providers and.consumers, highly trained and qualified professionals and barely schooled practitioners of many descriptions and a wide range of abilities.

Holism has, of course, always been integral to healing. Hippocrates emphasized the environmental causes and treatment of illness, and the importance of emotional factors and nutrition. And even a cursory reading of Chinese and Indian texts reveals the importance that these ancient healing traditions placed on the harmony between the individual and the social and natural world, on diet, self-care and self-regulation. Holism is emphasized now – at times, perhaps too stridently – to balance more recent technologically shaped tendencies to equate health care with the surgical and pharmacological treatment of specific disease entities and to ignore the shaping force of social and economic factors on health, to confuse, in Sir Williams Osler's words, the patient with his [or her] illness.

Most practitioners who describe themselves as holistic work independently. Pediatricians, family physicians, and internists may combine modalities in which they have not been formally certified or licensed – for example, psychotherapy, physical exercise, and nutrition – with those in which they have, while a nutritionist may offer advice on exercise and interpersonal relations as well as diet. Often as practitioners have become convinced of the utility of a wide range of techniques (and as the volume of their practice has increased) they have hired or gone into partnership with other professionals with different backgrounds and skills. For example, it has become increasingly

common for primary care physicians to hire massage therapists, nutritionists, health counselors, and acupuncturists
as auxiliary personnel, or for two or more non-medical
practitioners – a massage therapist, an acupuncturist, and a
psychologist – to form partnerships.

Sometimes such associations evolve into holistic health
centers. Equally often centers result from a common decision
by a group of practitioners, together with interested community members and patients, to create a new and different kind of
health care setting, one characterized by a professional
approach and interpersonal environment that attempts to heal
all participants.

Characteristics of holistic health centers

There is, however, no single model holistic health center, nor
ought there to be one. The programs that have evolved over the
last decade are as varied as the personalities and backgrounds,
the talents and needs of their founders, the staffs they have
attracted, the clients who have made use of their services, and
the geographical areas in which they are located. Most have
already undergone profound changes, and all, if they are to
remain – or become – responsive to their staffs' and clients'
changing needs, will have to continue to evolve. There are,
however, a number of characteristics which do help to define
and describe the ideal type of holistic health center.

1   *Though they do so in a variety of ways, holistic health
centers are concerned with developing comprehensive
programs which address the physical, psychological, and spiritual needs of those who come to them for help.* The Wholistic
Healing Centers, now a network of low cost, primary care clinics in suburbs, cities, and rural areas on the East Coast and in
the Midwest, began eleven years ago as a free clinic for low-
income people, staffed by volunteers and operating out of a
church basement in Springfield, Ohio. Its minister-founder,
Granger Westberg, hoped to restore the Christian Church's
healing mission, to infuse medical practice with meaning, and
to conserve resources by using the same building for two purposes (Tubesing 1979).

These clinics, which, according to Westberg stress "whole-ness rather than piety," emphasize God's – and the clin-ic's – total acceptance of each person and a hope for the sick that is at once theologically sound and biologically useful. Teams of ministers, nurses, and physicians work jointly with clients in initial planning sessions to help them formulate health programs that address psychological and spiritual as well as physical needs. The treatment they offer is a synthesis of allopathic medical care, pastoral counseling, and biofeedback, and is augmented by education in stress reduction, parent effec-tiveness training, yoga, meditation, and other physical and mental health practices.

At the Pain and Health Rehabilitation Center in Springfield, Missouri, C. Norman Shealy, a neurosurgeon who became dis-illusioned with the deleterious effects of drugs and the short-comings of surgery, has created a program that addresses the bodies, minds, and spirits of sufferers from chronic pain (1976). Shealy began ten years ago in a similar setting in LaCrosse, Wisconsin, with a fairly mechanistic approach. Transcutan-eous electrical nerve stimulation (TENS), facet rhizotomies, and behavior modification were his primary therapeutic modal-ities. Today he combines withdrawal from analgesics with diet, physical fitness, massage, biofeedback, TENS, and biogenics. This latter is a synthesis of progressive relaxation, autogenic training, Jungian therapy, and psychosynthesis, which is designed to help the practititioner to achieve the feeling of peace and acceptance that Shealy calls "spiritual attunement" as well as to relieve pain.

At the time that Westberg and Shealy were opening their clinics, O. Carl Simonton, a radiation oncologist in the United States Army, was beginning to study the therapeutic potential of the placebo response and of the faith and hope that are its constituents. After his discharge, he and his wife Stephanie Mathews-Simonton, opened the Cancer Counseling and Research Center in Fort Worth, Texas (1978). Their program, which works primarily with people who have widely dissemi-nated metastatic cancer, includes radiation therapy but relies to a large extent on procedures – visualization exercises, indi-vidual, family and group counseling in a supportive environ-ment – that stimulate the person's will to live and, with it, so far as they are able to tell, the body's immune response.

2 *Holistic health centers design health programs to meet the unique needs of each individual.* The lengthy meetings – "initial planning conferences" or "evaluations" – that are the first step in most programs generally produce a plan that includes ways to resolve the presenting problem, a summary of the client's long-term goals for health and well-being, and a strategy for achieving them.

A teenager with asthma who comes to a large and diverse program like the Wholistic Health and Nutrition Institute in Mill Valley, California, might receive a shot of epinephrine for her acute attack, but her planning conference would probably develop a program of withdrawal from antihistamines and bronchodilators. It might include stress reduction through biofeedback and relaxation exercises and a dietary change to eliminate foods that were allergenic for her. A longer term strategy to help her achieve greater self-confidence and independence would perhaps involve counseling with her family to remove the interpersonal binds that precipitate and perpetuate this kind of psychophysiological condition and a jogging clinic to help improve her vital capacity and feelings about her own body. A second youngster with asthma with a different psychophysiologic make-up might be treated quite differently.

3 *Holistic health centers preferentially use therapeutic approaches that mobilize the individual's capacity for self-healing and independence rather than pharmacological or surgical remedies that have negative side effects and tend to promote further dependence.* In all centers there is an emphasis on techniques like biofeedback, progressive relaxation, acupressure, guided imagery, yoga, and Tai Chi, which enable people to experience and then alter physical and emotional states that they had always regarded as beyond their control.

For example, at the Pain and Health Rehabilitation Center in Springfield and the Bresler Center in Los Angeles (Bresler and Trubo 1979), these modalities are used to help people quickly to reduce or withdraw from the high doses of analgesics on which they have been maintained for years.

4 *Holistic health centers emphasize education and self-care rather than treatment and dependence.* Practitioners tend to believe that each person is his or her best source of care, that

their job is to share rather than withhold and mystify their knowledge, to become "resources" rather than authorities. Like a growing number of clinicians who work in other settings, they tend to emphasize short-term problem oriented psychotherapy and common-sense behavioral prescriptions rather than psychodynamic analysis.

Almost all centers provide extensive brochures and introductory talks about their approach to health care and the techniques they use. The vast majority present a variety of classes to increase the well-being and supplement the coping skills of those who come to them for help. Stress reduction, parent effectiveness and assertiveness training, communication skills, yoga, transcendental meditation, and jogging are staples. In programs like the Kripalu Center in Western Massachusetts, the Holistic Health Center in Lexington, Kentucky, and the Himalayan Institute, a network of primary care clinics in which western medicine, yogic practice, and psychotherapy are synthesized, the techniques used in the clinical services are also taught in programs specifically designed for lay people.

Other groups, though not designed to provide the full range of clinical services (like the Berkeley Holistic Health Center, San Diego's Association for Holistic Health, and Interface in Brookline, Massachusetts), offer courses that are themselves a form of therapy. As one learns about visual retraining, massage, or meditation from a skilled teacher, one may indeed improve one's eyesight, relieve functional musculoskeletal problems, and reduce high blood pressure. These educational institutions are themselves closely tied to one or more holistic health centers with each serving as an adjunct to and source of referrals for the other.

5 *Holistic health centers treat those who come to them for help as members of families and social systems.* This enables practitioners to view their clients' symptoms as reactions to and communications within their familial or social situation as well as biological phenomena. As part of their intake process most centers make extensive inquiries, both in person and through questionnaires, into job satisfaction, community involvement, and psychosocial stress. In some centers members of the family are interviewed together, and clinicians can observe the way they relate to one another. A few programs like

Los Angeles' Learning for Health Center has a primary focus on therapeutic work with families, one or more of whose members is chronically ill. Others which work with people with chronic illness like Whole Health Associates in Newton, Massachusetts, the Pain and Rehabilitation Center and the Cancer Counseling and Research Center, are also eager to mobilize the strengths of other family members to support the afflicted individual or, more often, to work together to resolve patterns that may encourage one of them to remain in a "sick role." In fact, several residential centers which recognize the therapeutic potential of this approach offer reduced rates to the symptomatic person's spouse.

Programs for those who have psychophysiological problems that are not life-threatening or for people who are concerned with health promotion also encourage family participation. Counselors work with couples to help them to stop smoking or lose weight or to teach them how to massage one another.

6   *Holistic health centers view health as a positive state, not as the absence of disease, and emphasize health promotion and wellness.* This approach makes it possible for people who lack demonstrable organic pathology but feel poorly to enter holistic health programs, and encourages those who do have chronic organic disease to feel as well as they can within the limits set by the disease. Many centers offer courses to improve well-being by reducing stress and provide groups for people who want to stop smoking, lose weight, become more physically fit, or improve their communication with others. In many cases, the techniques that are used to promote better health are identical with those that are used to treat illness. At Oregon's Klamath Mental Health Center, for example, biofeedback is used to reduce stress and promote relaxation for those who simply want to feel more peaceful, more in control of their lives, as well as those who have such conditions as migraine headache, back pain, and hypertension.

Since John Travis (1977), a physician specializing in public health, first opened his Wellness Resource Center in Mill Valley, California, in 1974, "wellness" has become an influential concept, spurring the creation of programs like the Swedish Wellness Program at the Swedish Medical Center in Engelwood, Colorado, which have themselves become the models for dozens of other programs in hospitals and other work sites. Though Travis described a continuum between wellness and holistic medical and health programs (the former he maintained was oriented more toward prevention and education and depended almost exclusively, on client self-responsibility), his concept of wellness actually dovetailed nicely with the holistic approach. Indeed, many of the attitudes and approaches pioneered in wellness programs have been adopted by holistic health centers.

In wellness programs, individual counseling sessions and such standardized tests as Health Hazards Appraisals, Social Readjustment Rating Scales, and Wellness Inventories are used to help clients understand the relationship between their behaviors and their health, to see that what and how much they eat, smoke, and exercise, how they drive, the way they work, and how they get along with their families all affect the way they feel physically and emotionally. Together staff and clients review the factors that are likely to make them ill or to shorten their lives, and plan programs to eliminate or mitigate them.

7   *Though holistic centers emphasize the preeminent importance of careful, sensitive history-taking, and clinical examination and most use such conventional diagnostic methods as X-rays, blood chemistry, urinalysis, and psychological testing, some also include a variety of diagnostic techniques derived from other healing systems.* The Center for Traditional Acupuncture in Columbia, Maryland, the Bresler Center, and Whole Health Associates, for example, rely heavily on practitioners who have trained in both traditional Chinese and modern western medicine. In case conferences they compare and contrast findings obtained by Chinese pulse diagnosis and western laboratory analysis. Some program directors, including Evarts Loomis at the residential center Meadowlark in Hemet, California (Loomis and Paulson 1975), Norman Shealy and David Bresler are interested in bringing scientific rigor to the study of the alternative diagnostic procedures they use including iridology, pulse diagnosis, auricular diagnosis, and psychic diagnosis.

8   *Holistic health centers emphasize proper diet and exercise as cornerstones of healing.* Physicians at the Kripalu Center in

Western Massachusetts and at the Wholistic Health and Nutrition Institute use fasts or raw food diets or increased amounts of particular foods therapeutically. Increasing numbers of centers including the Springs Health Center in upstate New York and Commonweal in Bolinas, California, and Kripalu pay close attention to allergies to food and inhalants. The tests that they use suggest that these allergies are more prevalent and far more likely to precipitate or exacerbate a variety of illnesses than has previously been supposed.

Even centers which do not prescribe fasts or make use of the testing procedures of clinical ecology advise their clients to cut down on processed, refined, and preserved foods; on sugar, artificial sweeteners, colorings, and flavorings; to increase the amount of fiber, complex carbohydrates, and raw food in the diet; to eat somewhat less red meat and take stimulants like tea and coffee and depressants like alcohol in moderation. The meals they serve at parties or during workshops or residential sessions reflect these views.

Some programs emphasize the role that yoga or Tai Chi or indeed, running, may play in spiritual development as well as in improving physical and emotional health. Other centers like the Hills Sports and Fitness Center outside of Austin, Texas, are more concerned with the aerobic value of particular exercises. Many centers have ongoing "clinics" devoted to particular physical disciplines, and running or doing yoga with a client is sometimes an integral part of ongoing therapy.

9 *Holistic health centers maximize the therapeutic potential of the setting in which health care takes place.* The centers are generally both physically and interpersonally inviting and tend to inspire trust rather than fear or awe. Some, like Kripalu, the Pain and Health Rehabilitation Center, the Hills and Meadowlark are rural retreats where clients can experience a changed, more introspective relaxed way of life as well as a particular therapeutic regimen. Meadowlark in fact is consciously modeled on the ancient Greek healing temples which emphasized dreams and meditation as a source of healing for physical and emotional disability. Most centers are non-residential. A few like Westberg's Wholistic Health Centers occupy parts of such existing community institutions as churches and schools. Their design leans heavily toward open

spaces and attractively decorated, plant filled rooms.

Those who come for help are generally called clients rather than patients and are often encouraged to call staff members by their first names and to see the center as a place for education, volunteer work, and socializing as well as care in health and illness. Clients who do not have money often are able to barter services for health care and at least in one case, the Gesundheit Center near Washington, DC, they are cared for without any cost.

10 *Holistic health centers rely on an active partnership between care givers and consumers.* This connection is strongest in a program like the Eugene, Oregon, Community Health Education Center, which was started at the impetus of a broad-based neighborhood coalition supporting low-cost health care. This worker managed collective of physicians, nurses, health aides, and social workers charges minimal fees for comprehensive primary care – $15 for the first visit and $8.50 for the follow-ups – and is concerned with creating programs that respond directly to the felt needs of the community or for low-cost practical remedies to the problems that face them, such as child rearing, dietary management, physical fitness.

Connections also exist in programs in more affluent areas. Community people, including prominent local health care professionals, are included on boards of directors, and their demands, needs and advice shape the kinds of educational programs and health care techniques that are offered in the program.

11 *Holistic health centers include lay people and other professionals as well as MDs, DOs, PhDs, and RNs in the management of their centers.* Few programs have gone so far as the Community Health Education Center, a worker–managed collective in which all staff from physicians to licensed practical nurses are paid equally and participate equally in decision-making. However, virtually all centers make an active attempt to include nurses and massage therapists, receptionists, health counselors, and client volunteers in formulating policy and making day-do-day decisions about the center's operation.

12 *Holistic health centers provide an environment that is*

conducive to the personal growth of staff as well as clients. Informality of staff relations, the relative absence of hierarchical distinctions, the emphasis on cooperation and emotional sharing often makes these centers feel more like a family than a physician's office or a clinic. A high value is placed on sharing feelings and on staff members using their therapeutic talents and their emotional resources to help one another as well as their clients. Much attention is paid to forestalling the dangers of overwork, isolation, authoritarian behavior, and excessive self-criticism which seem to contribute to ''burnout'' and ''impairment'' in so many health care settings.

13   *Ongoing training of staff and of professionals in the community is an integral part of holistic health centers.* Such training is one means by which nonprofessional staff can acquire skills and change their position within the center. It offers a way for practitioners to expand their knowledge and tends to catalyze changes in the therapeutic program.

Many centers also serve as resources for local professionals who are interested in incorporating a more holistic approach – or new techniques – in their practice. A number of programs, including the Pain and Health Rehabilitation Center, the Himalayan Institute, the San Francisco-based East-West Academy of Healing Arts, and Los Angeles' Center for Integral Medicine, have week or month-long intensive courses and ongoing seminars for professionals. As they become more sophisticated, organizations are able to award continuing education credits for physicians and nurses.

Other groups like the Center for Traditional Acupuncture, the Himalayan Institute, and San Francisco's Nurse Consultants and Health Counselors are actively involved in training students in the health care professions, and several programs, including the Pain and Health Rehabilitation Center, Commonweal and Kripalu, and looking forward to instituting accredited rotations for medical students, interns, and residents.

14   *Holistic health centers are concerned with incorporating healing systems and healers indigenous to their areas into their work.* This is an act of ecological faith as well as a matter of good clinical sense. Centers in western states have consulted

with Native American healers and incorporated some of their rituals and herbs into their therapeutic programs. Centers in cities have made use of faith healers and curanderos, and rural centers throughout the country have readily included indigenous plants into their pharmacopoeia.

15   *Holistic health centers view illness as an opportunity for learning and change and are concerned with creating a context in which that kind of change can take place.* Even if it is not "natural" for western trained health professionals to regard illness as anything but an enemy, it is not difficult for them to realize that a flu or a bout of mononucleosis can be a sign of depression or that they can help a middle-aged executive to understand that a heart attack is a warning to slow down. It is far more difficult for centers which deal with people with chronic and often fatal illnesses to continue to help their clients wrest a sense of personal meaning from the illness that may soon kill them, for counselors and physicians to keep themselves from blame and self-doubt when their clients die. Work like this takes place in the Cancer Counseling and Research Center, the Pain and Health Rehabilitation Center, Whole Health Associates, and many other, newer programs. It requires a considerable amount of time and mutual support, as well as extraordinary honesty and is a hallmark of many holistic centers.

16   *Though the absence of funds has handicapped research efforts, holistic health centers are beginning to study themselves and their work with clients.* Anthropological studies of one Northern California center (Mattson 1982) has already been completed as has a second at the Berkeley Psychosomatic Clinic. Most programs are keeping careful records and many are trying to move beyond anecdotal to systematic studies. The Pain and Health Rehabilitation Center, Commonweal, and the Cancer Counseling and Research Center have all been collecting follow-up data on their patients for some time. The results are preliminary and in all cases the clients are their own controls. Still, these programs report high rates of success in reducing pain, amount of medication used, and surgery (Gordon, Jaffe, and Bresler 1983). In the case of the Cancer Counseling program, the productive life of a number of patients

with widely disseminated metastatic disease has been prolonged well beyond statistical probability and the expectations
of their physicians.

The future of holistic health centers

As knowledge about a holistic approach to health and illness
becomes more widespread, increased numbers of clients with a
greater variety of problems are coming to the centers. Many
centers are responding by changing to meet the needs of their
clients. A program like the Pain and Health Rehabilitation
Center, which originally restricted itself to working with people with chronic pain, has now begun to apply its therapeutic
approach to people who are simply stressed, and centers that
initially worked with the "worried well" have begun to welcome the challenge of dealing with people who have serious
illnesses.

The interest and the demand is widespread enough to stimulate Granger Westberg to plan for Wholistic Health Centers in a
half dozen more cities, and intense enough to encourage
existing centers like Lexington's Holistic Health Centre
toward a continual expansion of their services.

Leslie Kaslof's authoritative *Wholistic Dimensions in
Healing* (1978) noted approximately fifty holistic health
centers, now, five years after he compiled his listing, there are
certainly several hundred programs which would define themselves as holistic, most of which may be legitimately classified
as such. In the Washington, DC area alone, three have opened
in the last year. There are also, within the context of hospitals,
corporations, etc., several hundred "wellness" programs.
These generally offer employees a range of health promotion
activities including counseling designed to explore the relations between individual behaviors and health, and programs
designed to reduce stress and improve fitness.

At the same time that the model is being developed in holistic
health centers it is also being applied in alternatives to conventional services that confine their work to people at particular
stages of the life cycle, and in programs created by and for
women. Comprehensive home birth programs, like Lewis
Mehl's Berkeley Family Health Center, have offered family

counseling, prenatal care, and instruction in natural remedies as well as in natural childbirth. Centers for runaway young people and group foster homes are beginning to pay more attention to the food they serve young people, to discuss exercise and health care as well as living places and schools to suggest meditation or relaxation exercises as well as family therapy. In Phoenix, physicians and psychologists who are disciples of the Indian teacher, Yogi Bhajan, have created a comprehensive non-drug residential detoxification program for young addicts which combines Kundalini yoga, meditation, nutrition, and an intense group therapeutic experience, and in Houston, Texas, plans have been made for a multi-million dollar Holistic Health and Rehabilitation Center, a city and county funded program for young people with psychosocial and drug related problems. At the other end of the life cycle, services for the elderly modeled on Berkeley's SAGE (Senior Actualization and Growth Experience) (Dychtwald 1978) and hospices and other projects for the dying like the San Francisco Bay Area's Shanti program have adopted a holistic approach (Garfield 1979).

Women's programs like the Berkeley Women's Health Collective and San Francisco's Haight Ashbury Women's Medical Clinic combine general medical and gynecological care with an emphasis on prevention, natural remedies, and consciousness raising groups. For several years in Dorchester, Massachusetts, minority women who ran the Columbia Point Alcoholism Program provided a comprehensive residential program for Hispanic and Black women and their children. The program used fasts to detoxify alcoholics and combined instruction about natural foods and herbs, rhythmic breathing, physical exercise, and meditation with education, child care, rehabilitation counseling, and social services (Gordon 1978).

The model that has been created in holistic centers and applied in other alternative services has also been integrated into the mainstream of health care. Donald Ardell, editor of the *American Journal of Health Planning*, notes that Health Systems Agencies, established under the Health Planning and Resource Development Act of 1974, are currently involved in providing technical assistance to health promotion and wellness programs in schools, the work place, hospitals, and neighborhood health centers. One of the most active of these, the Madison, Wisconsin, Health Planning Council, has, for example, helped a small hospital in Columbus, Wisconsin, to create a wellness program for employees that includes running, nutritional classes, yoga, transcendental meditation, cross-country skiing, and stress management (Ardell 1980).

Government bureaucracies, eager to practice some of what they preach, have also begun to pay attention to improving their employees' health. At the Public Health Service's Center for Disease Control in Atlanta, 70 per cent of the 2,200 employees are participating in health education programs which, like the Wellness Resource Center, begin by identifying physical and psychological risk factors in each person's life.

Though there is little information so far on holistic health centers in the professional literature, they are being discussed in workshops at meetings of the American Holistic Medical Association and the American Holistic Nurses Association. At public conferences across the country, groups like the Association for Holistic Health, the Himalayan Institute, the Center for Integral Medicine, the East–West Academy of Healing Arts, and the Institute for the Study of Human Knowledge are presenting these programs and the techniques used in them to audiences which not uncommonly exceed one to two thousand professionals and lay people.

The effect of all these activities is now being felt in the schools of the health care professions. Departments of behavioral medicine, family practice, community medicine, and psychiatry, schools of nursing and public health, are sponsoring lecture series and elective courses in holistic approaches to health and medicine. Techniques used in holistic health centers – acupuncture, relaxation therapies, autogenic training, visual imagery, massage – are increasingly being incorporated into the practice of more conventional medical settings and larger scale experiments in adopting the holistic approach to the clinic and hospital are under way. At Yale Medical School, for example, a study of the use of guided imagery in the treatment of cancer which the Simontons pioneered at the Cancer Counseling and Rehabilitation Center, is under way. And in Boston, Dr Jonathan Lieff and his colleagues are bringing a holistic approach to the treatment of chronic illness to the Lemuel Shattuck Hospital.

To make available these and other opportunities to medical students and house officers, Raymond Rosenthal and I have compiled a Directory of some 160 distinguished health care professionals who have agreed to act as preceptors (direct supervisors) and resource persons (advisors) to students. Many of those listed are currently directing and working in holistic health centers. Others are involved in clinical work, research on administrative activities which emphasize this approach.

With all of this activity much still needs to be changed, within existing centers and in the relationship between centers and the larger medical and non-medical community. For example, some practitioners who call themselves holistic, and indeed some facilities that purport to be holistic health centers, seem as parochial as the hospitals and subspecialists they criticize. There is nothing holistic about allowing poorly trained personnel to practice or about claiming that diet or chiropractic or acupuncture or homeopathy can cure every illness.

Training, and an increased emphasis on quality control, are needed. For the present it seems important to achieve a balance between openness to unconventional healers and regulation of unscrupulous practitioners who flourish at the fringe of medicine and capitalize on the despair of prospective patients.

It is also imperative to study carefully the individual techniques used in the holistic health center and the approach itself. Established research methodologies like the double blind study may well be inappropriate for evaluating techniques like relaxation therapies, visualization, and yoga, which depend for their efficacy on the active informed participation of patients. We need methodologies that can accommodate subtle variations in individualized treatment as well as the synergistic effect of the combination of treatments that are being developed in holistic health centers, and, indeed, the therapeutic effect of the setting on staff who work in it. And some of our research must be directed not to controlling for these effects but to determining how to maximize them.

There is also the danger that holistic health centers will continue to be primarily a luxury for the wealthy, that their doctrine of self-help and individual responsibility will be perverted to public neglect. The present prevalence of holistic health centers in upper middle class areas has more to do with physicians' preferences and economic self-interest than it does with the wishes or capabilities of patients. One of Rev. Granger Westberg's most successful centers is in a lower middle class suburb and Dr Walt Stoll's Holistic Health Centre opened in a working-class community. My own experience in community-based programs with inner-city black youth suggests that, given the proper therapeutic context, they are quite willing to change their diet or do relaxation exercises or have family therapy – if they believe it will clear up their acne or relieve their anxiety.

At present, however, virtually all holistic health centers are still private for-profit practices based on a fee-for-service model. This helps to restrict health care to an elite minority and may it itself be inimical to a holistic practice.

Most health promotion and disease prevention strategies, as well as many of the modalities used in the holistic approach, are not covered by existing insurance policies or by Medicare or Medicaid. Even in the case of patients who are wealthy – or are adequately covered by insurance – the fee-for-service model still shapes and skews care. In a holistic as well as a biomedical practice, fee-for-service care provides economic encourage-ment for elaborate diagnostic tests and time consuming thera-pies and procedures. Though these may sometimes be useful, they tend to work in opposition to the kind of self-exploration and self-help that are at the heart of the holistic approach. This pattern of reimbursement also tends to encourage providers to conceptualize their patients' conditions and the services they offer according to conventional diagnostic and therapeutic categories. Finally, since they are only reimbursed when they are providing care, it exerts a subtle pressure on providers to keep their patients dependent.

If holistic practice is not to degenerate under the weight of fee-for-service financial imperatives, alternative means of financing must be developed. These strategies must give pro-viders economic incentives to help their patients stay healthy at the same time that they guarantee ready access to health care. They must also recognize that holistic health care should strike a balance between the center's need for clinical freedom and self-governance and the community's need for responsive services and oversight.

It is time to create model holistic programs in a variety of communities, to assess whether a combination of health pro-motion and public education and of western and alternative medicine can meet people's needs more effectively and less expensively than the present system. Such experimental programs would be designed to provide comprehensive health care on a prepaid basis to a particular community or neighborhood. They should be compared in long-term longitudinal studies, both with more conventional prepaid health care and the standard fee-for-service system. Their evaluation should include, in an analysis of costs and benefits, measures of patient satisfaction, quality of life and psychological change, as well as more conventional assessments of morbidity and mortality.

Conclusion

As the numbers of holistic health centers increase, as the centers themselves continue to grow and develop, their attitudes toward health and healing, the techniques they use, and the way they synthesize them will continue to be incorporated into the mainstream of medical care and of health promotion efforts. At the same time there will be tendencies to dilute or pervert the approach, to use it to justify neglect of public health or to appropriate the techniques used in the centers, while neglecting the interpersonal context in which they are used. In the years to come the centers must continue to grow and develop, to insist on the spirit as well as the letter of their practice.

References

Ardell, D.B. (1980) The Physical Disciplines and Health. In A. Hastings, J. Fadiman and J.S. Gordon (eds) *Health for the Whole Person: The Complete Guide to Holistic Medicine*. New York: Bantam.

Bresler, D.E. and Trubo, R. (1979) *Freedom from Pain*. New York: Simon & Schuster.

Dychtwald, K. (1978) *Bodymind*. New York: Jove.

Eisenberg, L. (1977) Psychiatry and Society: A Sociobiological Synthesis. *New England Journal of Medicine* 296(16): 903–10.

Engel, G.L. (1977) The Need for a New Medical Model: A Challenge to Biomedicine. *Science* 196: 129–36.

Garfield, C.A. (1979) *Stress and Survival: The Emotional Realities of Life-Threatening Illness*. St Louis: Mosby.

Gordon, J.S. (1978) *Final Report of the Special Study on Alternative Services*. Report to the President of the President's Commission on Mental Health. Washington, DC, US Govt Printing Office.

——(1980) Holistic Health Centers. In A. Hastings, J. Fadiman and J.S. Gordon (eds) *Health for the Whole Person: The Complete Guide to Holistic Medicine*. New York: Bantam.

——(1981) The Paradigm of Holistic Medicine. In A. Hastings, J. Fadiman and J.S. Gordon (eds) *Health for the Whole Person: The Complete Guide to Holistic Medicine*. New York: Bantam.

Gordon, J.S., Jaffe, D., and Bresler, D. (eds) (1984) *Mind, Body and Health: Towards an Integral Medicine*. New York: Human Sciences Press.

Kaslof, L.J. (ed.) (1978) *Wholistic Dimensions in Healing*. New York: Doubleday.

Loomis, E.G. and Paulson, J.S. (1975) *Healing for Everyone*. New York: Hawthorne.

Mattson, P.H. (1982) *Holistic Health in Perspective*. Palo Alto: Mayfield.

Shealy, N.C. (1976) *The Pain Game*. Millbrae, California: Celestial Arts.

Simonton, O.C., Matthews-Simonton, S., and Creighton, J. (1978) *Getting Well Again*. Los Angeles: J.P. Tarcher.

Smuts, J.C. (1926) *Holism and Evolution*. New York: Macmillan.

Travis, J.W. (1977) *Wellness Workbook*. Mill Valley, California: Wellness Resource Center.

Tubesing, D.A. (1979) *The Wholistic Health Center*. New York: Human Science Press.

Listing of resources

American Holistic Medical Association
6932 Little River Turnpike
Annandale, Virginia 22003

Rudolph M. Ballentine MD
Director of Therapy Programs
Himalayan Institute
RD 1, Box 88
Honesdale, Pennsylvania 18431

Ballentine, R. (1978) *Diet and Nutrition*. Honesdale, Pa.; Himalayan Press.

Swami Ajaya (ed.) (PhD.)
"Holistic Therapy."
Meditational Therapy.
Honesdale, Pa; Himalayan Press.

David E. Bresler PhD, CA
Director
Bresler Center Medical Group
12401 Wilshire Blvd. Suite 280
Los Angeles, California 90025

Bresler, D.E. and Trubo, R.
(1979) *Free Yourself from
Pain*. New York: Simon &
Schuster.

Dianne M. Connelly, PhD,
MAC
Founder and Practitioner
The Centre for Traditional
Acupuncture
108 American City Bldg.
Columbia, Maryland 21044

Connelly, D. (1975) *Traditional
Acupuncture: The Law of the
5 Elements*.
The Centre for Traditional
Acupuncture.

Connelly, D., editor and
contributor, *The Journal of
Traditional Acupuncture*.

Ted Edwards MD
Hills Medical Sports Complex
4615 W. Bee-Caves Road
Austin, Texas 78746

Edwards, T. and Lau, B. (1982)
*Weight Loss to Super Well-
ness*. Hills Medical Sports
Complex.

James S. Gordon MD
Aurora Associates Inc.
1140 Connecticut Ave. NW
Washington, DC 20036

Hastings, A., Fadiman, J., and
Gordon, J. (1980) *Health for
the Whole Person: The Complete Guide to Holistic
Medicine*. New York: Bantam.

Rosenthal, R., Gordon, J. (1984)
*New Directions in Medicine:
A Directory of Learning
Opportunities*. Aurora
Associates Inc.

Richard Ingrasci MD, MPH
Co-Director
Whole Health Associates
70 Phillips St.
Watertown, Massachusetts
02172

Health Dialogue, a monthly
column for *New Age* magazine
(1980–   ).

Dennis T. Jaffe PhD
Co-Director
Learning for Health Center
1314 Westwood Blvd. Suite 107
Los Angeles, California 90024

Jaffe, D. (1980) *Healing from
Within: Becoming the
Architect of Your Health*.
New York: Knopf.

Jonathan Lieff MD
Lemuel Shattuck Hospital
170 Morton Street
Jamaica Plain, Massachusetts
02130

Evarts G. Loomis. MD, FACS
Executive Director
Friendly Hills Fellowship
26126 Fairview Ave.
Hemet, California 92343

Loomis, E.G. and Paulson, J.S.
(1975) *Healing for Everyone*.
New York: Hawthorne.

Lewis E. Mehl MD
Center for Research on Birth
and Human Development
2340 Ward St., Room 105
Berkeley, California 94705

Jeffrey Migdow MD
Homoeopathy
Kripalu Center for Holistic

Health
PO Box 120–1
Summit Station, Pennsylvania
17979

Migdow, J. *Kripalu Yoga Quest*, vol. 4, no 1, Kripalu Yoga Institute.

Norman Shealy MD, PhD
Shealy Institute
1919 S. Freemont
Springfield, Missouri 65804

Shealy, C.N. (1977) *90 Days to Self-Health*. New York: Dial Press.

O. Carl Simonton MD
Cancer Counseling and Research Center
6060 N. Central Expressway

Suite 140
Dallas, Texas 75206

Simonton, C., Matthews-Simonton, S., and Creighton, J. (1978) *Getting Well Again*. New York: Bantam.

Walter Stoll Jr, MD
Medical Director
Holistic Health Center
1412 N. Broadway
Lexington, Kentucky 40505

Granger Westberg DD
Wholistic Health Centers, Inc.
137 S. Garfield St.
Hinsdale, Illinois 60521

Tubesing, D.A. *The Wholistic Health Center*. New York: Human Sciences Press.

Nine

Defining health and reorganizing medicine

J. Warren Salmon

Out of the critique of scientific medicine have come suggestions for a reformulation of medical conceptions and theories. Proponents of such a reorientation maintain that demographic, cultural, and economic changes over coming decades will eventually necessitate expansion of the domain of health care institutions. People assuming greater responsibility for their own health through lifestyle alterations is also seen as a significant megatrend. These proponents believe that mainstream medicine will soon undergo a revitalization with an infusion of new preventive technologies; clinical applications from a host of new and alternative therapeutics; and revolutionary findings from research on the mind and brain.

The arrival of this new theory and practice of medicine may await a fuller understanding of what constitutes human health, but acceptance by the dominant health care system is generally foreseen given the "paradigm shift" resulting from evolving scientific discoveries and changing human thought in the population. In other words, the hopes, aspirations, and ideas within this perspective on health and healing are presumed to be in themselves a force for positive social change, reflected in the "new consciousness." Ferguson (1980: 241) views the "impending transformation of medicine [as] a window to the transformation of all institutions."

This short depiction is a composite rendering of what may be gleaned from holistic health and consciousness literature and conferences over the last several years. It characterizes a viewpoint of the "New Age" movement, which has become an influential subculture in the US. Optimism usually outweighs evidence for their claims regarding the future social and cultural scene. Nevertheless, the point can be made that as variations on this theme are expressed more widely, this social vision may assume greater ideological meaning and gradually receive wider attention. *Megatrends* accords favor to similar possible directions for health (Naisbett 1982). These perspectives and prospects for change bring with them calls from advocates for various alternative systems of medicine who seek greater legitimacy for their respective theories and practices. Together they hope to influence, and be a part of, the "new medicine" (Carlson 1975a, 1975b).

This chapter reviews and analyzes definitions of health offered from sources within the established health care system, contrasting them to some of what the more holistic oriented writers suggest. Broader social, ecological, and cosmological parameters to the concept of health are examined. Secondly, the "paradigm shift" in medicine is explored, relating back to points made previously about the nature of health. Here I briefly describe some implications from the "new physics" and how consciousness is believed to impact health and healing.

This most important discussion about the nature of health is considered in light of certain political economic developments in health and health care. The social definition of health (what constitutes its generation and restoration) takes on great significance today given conditions of escalating costs and questionable effectiveness of the respective health care systems in the United States and United Kingdom. Corporate and government strategies for restructuring the American delivery system render these deliberations more than a mere intellectual concern. Moreover, the increasing proprietization of health care institutions by nationwide profit-seeking entities is bringing about both managerial and technological innovations in the delivery of care. Over the next twenty years, these changes are likely to profoundly alter the content of medical services. The social control implications here may not be conspicuous if it appears as though improved services and cost efficiency can be promised for people with the ability to pay.

Arguments for enlarging the paradigm of scientific medicine are thus not abstract, inconsequential, or immaterial. There is an urgent need for greater popular awareness and critical discussion to assure more democratic determination of health services and changed social and ecological conditions for health. Such debates representing conflicting perceptions and values are characteristic of periods of social struggle, marking the transformation of existing social institutions. Challenges to the ideological hegemony of scientific medicine have made the contradictions within its organizational form more readily apparent (McKinlay 1984). However, any new epistemology of medicine will be formulated within the economic and cultural framework of the health care system and larger society. Thus, it is important to note how reconceptualizations of health, healing, and human existence may conform to and conflict with changing dominant thinking.

The definition problem of health

The concept of health is central to the understanding, evaluation, and advancement of any system of medicine. It is crucial to specifying the objectives of health care practitioners.

Most definitions of health under scientific medicine have assumed that it, like disease, is simply located in the body, and that its experience by a specific person is generally isolated from social life and larger forces. Health is usually seen to be experienced subjectively as an unshared individual process, even though it is created and recreated through objective events and relationships with one's external reality. While practitioners may recognize that these variously viewed and experienced events and relationships carry a personal reality to them, other thinkers claim there is much more to them (Bohm and Weber 1983; Dossey 1983). According to this latter view, there is an intimate connection between the individual's experience of health and the vast complexity of one's immediate family, work, and social networks; community setting; and the larger ecology (Hastings, Fadiman, and Gordon 1980). Some modern investigators of the mind now suggest what mystics and religious thinkers have identified centuries ago as the cosmological connection to the inner-self. These thoughts have become intertwined within current discussions on the definition of health as consideration is given to what previous civilizations and cultures viewed as the spiritual dimensions to health and illness before western biomedicine (Sobel 1979).

Scientific medicine, with its focus on disease symptomatology, assumes a state of health in the individual when its extensive clinical findings appear within normal ranges (Toulmin 1975). This narrow clinical perspective of biomedicine does not always regard illness behavior as important (Engel 1977). This is not to say physicians in practice do not maintain a sensitivity to patient well-being (Moser 1980), but that the orientation of western biomedicine tends toward an engineering or mechanical approach for repair of the human machine (Renaud 1975).

In broadening this, the World Health Organisation in 1947 provided the most widely used definition: "Health is the complete state of physical, mental, and social well-being, not merely the absence of disease." Primarily speaking to what *ought* to be, this definition offers wide interpretation.

One of the most influential thinkers on the subject has been Rene Dubos, who described health as an adaptation to the environment: "a modus vivendi enabling imperfect men to achieve a rewarding and not too painful existence while they cope with an imperfect world" (1968: 67). In an earlier work he emphasized host resistance, recognizing that "states of health are the expressions of the success or failure experienced by the organism in its effort to respond adaptively to environmental challenges" (Dubos 1965: 12). He described health as "the power to live a full, adult, living, breathing life in close contact with what I love – the earth and the wonders thereof" (Dubos 1965: 351). His perspective provides for a multicausal view of disease where internal biological, along with other human factors, govern the response of the individual to specific agents of disease, whether microbial, chemical, radiation, or whatever. He sees medicine constantly changing to confront disease, but never completely producing health: "The concept of perfect and positive health is a utopian creation of the mind. It cannot become reality because man will never be so perfectly adapted to his environment that his life will not involve struggles, failures, and sufferings" (Dubos 1965: 346). This struggle and adaptation dynamic appears in many definitions. Concerned with social structural elements of modern industrial societies and human autonomy, Illich sees health as: "the ability to adapt to changing environments, to growing up and to aging, to healing when damaged, to suffering, and to peaceful expectation of death. Health designates a process by which each person is responsible" (1976: 271). Unlike health practitioners, he argues for greatly reducing the province of medicine:

> Healthy people are those who live in healthy homes on a healthy diet in an environment equally fit for birth, growth, healing, and dying; they are sustained by a culture that enhances the conscious acceptance of limits to population, of aging, of incomplete recovery and ever imminent death. Healthy people need minimal bureaucratic interference to mate, give birth, share the human condition, and die.
>
> (Illich 1976: 272)

Given the complexities of human biology and social life, what then can be usefully, or appropriately, modified by health care practitioners? There is a wide range of interventions proposed by advocates of various alternative systems of medicine. These stem from a broader conception of health beyond the biological.

Most holistic health care responds to concerns for fitness, wellness, prevention, risk reduction, etc. For the most part though its major therapeutic interventions tend to principally focus upon the "internal balancing" of the person with greater participation by the patient in the process of treatment. In contrast to the women's health and community health movements, holistic advocates have generally played down the vast and ambiguous external forces about the individual, excepting the more metaphysical interpretations and some concern for the ecology. Drawing from South African Jan Christian Smuts (1926) practitioners of a gamut of various therapeutic modalities interject a triune nature of body, mind, and spirit in the concept of health. With roots in humanistic psychology, Maslow's hierarchy of needs is usually implied in the attainment of health (Maslow 1962). As with scientific medical physicians, alternative practitioners have felt practically constrained in making many interventions outward into the realm of the social world (Berliner and Salmon 1980); however, their attempts to address the "whole person" (where these therapies in fact do so) provide for a fuller conception of human functioning. Frequently aspects of personal growth and self-realization are incorporated (Berkeley Holistic Health Center 1978; LaPatra 1978; Albright and Albright 1980).

The ideology of the New Age movement emphasizes personal upgrading and self-improvement, thus influencing individual responsibility for health and well-being (Ferguson 1980). Ardell coined the phrase "high-level wellness" as:

> a lifestyle-focused approach designed for the purpose of pursuing the highest level of health within your capability. A wellness lifestyle is dynamic or ever-changing . . . an integrated lifestyle in that you incorporate some approach or aspect of each wellness dimension (self-responsibility, nutritional awareness, stress management, physical fitness, and environmental sensitivity). (Ardell 1977: 65)

The notion of "choice" over one's state of health (and disease) has been emphasized within holistic circles. It is constantly suggested that a sick person must utilize personal capacities and potentials to achieve an awareness of responsibility, choice, and control over his or her placement on the "health-illness continuum" (Travis 1977). In vogue today are health hazard appraisals and other self-assessments to heighten awareness of deleterious health behaviors and assist in changing them. Stress-management protocols, prospective medicine, and a variety of self-care approaches are also popular, as utilized in conventional medical settings too (Flynn 1980). These health education tools and interventions are based upon the dictum that the individual must exert greater responsibility for health – an easier set of tasks for the "worried well" of middle-age and middle class than for other social groups. This social stratum of course has the discretionary income to buy these services from entrepreneurs who have turned a cosmic ecological concern into a sales package marketed to aid coping with a stressful social existence.

Not so coincidentally, this set of endeavors resonates with government and corporate calls for individuals to change their lifestyles. These purchasers of medical care for public beneficiaries and employees and their families are seeking to lessen dependence on medical professionals to potentially reduce cost escalation in medical care (Berliner and Salmon 1979). With individuals being willing to pay out-of-pocket for newly styled services, institutionally guaranteed benefits need not be paid for by employers. To the extent that the populace believes health problems result mainly from personal behaviors, demands for health care as a basic right can be, and in fact are being, undermined in this period of economic contraction (Crawford 1977). This ideological notion serves a political use in justifying federal cutbacks and instituting greater cost-sharing. In other words, why should public monies be used to provide medical care to people who are not taking better care of themselves?

This lifestyles ideology has taken grip in the public mind. It was popularized by the late John Knowles of the Rockefeller Foundation (1976) and by the Federal reports (US Dept of Health, Education and Welfare), such as the *Forward Plan for Health - 1977–1981* (1976) and *Healthy People* (1979). In holistic circles, some ill-informed psychologizing neglects established multiple causation for specific diseases. This often misplaces emphasis in health maintenance on individual attitudes and behaviors (Sontag 1977; Simonton 1978). While not denying people's contributing to their own disease susceptibility, the point should be readily recognized that such a premise supports public policy which exculpates corporate responsibility for occupational and environmental health problems. At this time it is no social accident that the shift away from governmental responsibility for health proceeds in tandem with laying blame on the individual for illness. Popular support for a more balanced ecology and safer jobs is often challenged and undermined with this ideology.

Relatedly, Kelman (1975) sees the definition problem of health as vital to the directions of formulating health care policy. Taking the perspective from the sociology of knowledge, he argues for an analytical understanding of the social and historical context in which ideas about health arise, gain favor, or lose it. He maintains that the objectification of the person in modern capitalist society (i.e. becoming an object of corporate production) has serious health consequences, both psychological and physical. Kelman urges adoption of a "new paradigm" that recognizes health behavior in its proper societal context, with the focus largely on its socially determined aspects. Drawing from Piaget, he offers a definition with two fundamental and conflicting dimensions: experiential health referring to "intrinsically defined organismic integrity, whereas functional health refers to extrinsically defined organismic integrity" (within the latter the person has little say about his or her health). Kelman sees functional health as the purpose of health care planning in the US. Defining health in functional terms offers an explicit, empirical, and operational thrust to health policy, which enables expensive medical care resources to be diverted away from the economically unproductive (e.g. the poor, unemployed, aged, disabled, etc.). The policy directions pursued by the Reagan and Thatcher administrations to restrict expansion of medical care have given weight to this assessment. More pointedly, corporate discussions of rationing medical care resources (Goldbeck 1978) provoke an even greater concern about government policy initiatives to limit expenditures on medical care as well as public health (Mechanic 1978, 1979; Evans 1983; Fry 1983). The philosophical underpinnings related to the purpose of scientific medicine have held a long standing moral commitment to the preservation of life. Lately though policy analysts are building careers on the systematic design of such rationing schemes for expensive care, while a little more than a decade ago the topic would have been morally reprehensible in both Britain's National Health Service and the US (Aaron and Schwartz 1984).

During economic retrenchment, it seems logical for the sick to be scapegoated as the "cause" of their poor health status. This insidious social current parallels what can be seen in the division between the old and young (Estes 1979). As with the declared "crisis" of US Social Security System, the "health problem" has been socially constructed. The highly publicized "cost crisis" defines and interprets the need for social change, with dominant ideologies affecting our thinking about health, health care, and paradigm formulations. As large numbers of people, particularly those in important opinion-making positions, begin to act as if these conceptions are connected to concrete social phenomena, policy can be reshaped to appear as "progress" (Estes 1982).

The fact remains that the corporate class views the government-subsidized "non-productive" segments of the population as a major fiscal drain on the US economy. While not denying there is an empirical reality to what the individual can do, we should be aware that the victim-blaming tendency of current social policy is attempting to hold people accountable for their external predicament when unfortunately they are not empowered in the first place to alter it (Minkler 1983). It is vital that the evolving social definition of health does not erroneously assume that individuals create the fullness of their life conditions and social opportunities (Dreitzel 1971).

In light of Kelman's argument, it is interesting to review the predominant definition that has been used in medical sociology: Parsons states that health is "the state of optimal capacity of an individual for the effective performance of the roles and tasks for which he has been socialized" (Parsons 1972: 117). This implies that ability to perform is the sole requisite of health, leading Kelman to point out that: "If the performance of one's work is itself pathogenic (coal mining, asbestos processing, textile manufacturing, etc.), Parsons' definition identifies the result as illness only when it results in the absence from work, or, generally the incapacity to perform as socialized" (Kelman 1975: 636). In a similar vein Smith notes that:

> The role-performance model provides a minimal conception of health. Evidently persons able to perform adequately in their occupational roles may fail to achieve the self-actualization of Maslow's model or the adaptive facility of Dubos'. They may also fall short of the clinical model in that they may be physically ill even though able to fulfill their central roles.   (Smith 1981: 46)

In sum, it can be seen that functional health, though limited and servant to productive value, has overshadowed the experiential dimension – how the individual comes to view and work at his or her own well-being.

Social and environmental origins of disease

For over a century public health and epidemiology have been concerned with the social and environmental aspects of the onset and treatment of illness. In the 1840s, Rudolf Virchow, later the father of modern pathology, concluded that social, economic, and political factors had a great deal to do with causing a typhus epidemic, as did the biological and physical factors (Ackerknecht 1953). Virchow called for measures such as free public education, separation of church and state, higher wages, progressive taxation, cultural autonomy for national minorities, agricultural collectives, and full employment to reduce the susceptibility of the population to disease (Galdston 1952). He and other social medicine physicians saw the spread of disease as dependent upon class and social position. Social medicine, and the subsequent, though less-radical sanitary reform movement, were based upon the premise that society had an obligation to protect and enhance the health of its members (Rosen 1958). During the later years of the 1870s and 1880s the germ theory of disease and the theory of specific etiology (single causation) emerged in France and Germany (Ackerknecht 1968). They became the means for constructing new conceptions of disease and health, which became and remain basic supports of scientific medicine. With the practical successes of medicine in treating infectious diseases, germ theory, and the single etiology became the principal way of understanding disease causation (Berliner and Salmon 1980). The result was a tendency to downplay social and environmental factors and focus on more limited concerns that medicine could more easily remedy. As mentioned previously, the "non-scientific" spiritual realm of health and illness was neglected, and even stigmatized, in the subsequent development of modern biomedicine.

Over time, scientific medicine took on characteristics in its form and content from the larger economic system and has in some ways legitimated capitalist economic development (Navarro 1976; Waitzkin 1978; McKinlay 1984). Early capitalism heralded the individual, and scientific medicine integrated a model of healing that diagnosed illness as biological disease in the individual and individually prescribed treatment. As such its constructs filter the experiences of practitioners and patients alike. If one agrees with the critics of scientific medicine, it has offered a peculiar distortion in this process. The rationality of "science" that also served as the basis of scientific management (Braverman 1974) provided for the continual search for biological sources of disease, focusing away from fuller consideration of its linkages to social development (Eyer 1984).

Yet medicine has not just been an economic mode of production (Berliner 1983). Due to its particular human relationships and its healing tasks, the institution of modern medicine has possessed a relative autonomy within modern society up until the present era. Tied together in the complex social history of medicine have been the meanings and values assigned to healing; the power and domination of the medical profession; the range of political and economic forces that have shaped health care delivery; and the ideological and political ends that this form of medicine has served (Wright and Treacher 1983). Given this relative autonomy across history, it is crucial to anticipate the probable emphasis of a "new medicine" given changes urged by the corporate class for the "health maintenance" of its workforce; the reductions of services to the less fortunate; and the industrialization of medicine brought on by nationwide proprietary providers (Salmon 1984).

Individual or collective health

While broader social aspects of disease have been relatively unexplored and unincorporated in present medical practice, public health and social epidemiology have indicated differences in the occurrence, severity, and length of specific illnesses based upon a person's income, race, sex, age, and especially class (Susser and Watson 1971). The pressing problems of chronic diseases in advanced western societies have led to multi-factorial explanations for disease occurrence, with more numerous concrete social, occupational, and environmental linkages delineated in studies. The separation between medicine and public health; the relative political weakness of the latter; and the difficulty in methodologically demonstrating the causative nature to larger social, economic, and political factors have all influenced thinking and planning for our population's health.

Disease attacks human groups, as is obvious in epidemics of

infectious disease over history. This social reality seems to have been forgotten in the recent ontological reinterpretation of the individual in medicine (Wartofsky 1975). Even with chronic diseases today, epidemiological investigations vividly portray the nature and course of disease being a function of a collectivity of people (Brenner 1973; Waldron and Eyer 1975: Eyer 1977; Berkman and Syme 1979). The economic cycle and social groupings proscribe disease patterns. A population group's work, social relations, immediate environment and habitat, values and views of social life, the world and the universe are also contributory to their health status. For a complexity of reasons, these larger social interconnections of disease are inadequately understood in modern society. The orientation of scientific medicine and the evolved structure of health services has constrained a more thorough conception of our collective health, besides providing barriers to its investigation in practice (Totman 1979). The lack of a broader health mandate in public policy has also placed an ideological constriction on our thinking about health.

With recent concern over social stressors and ecological degradation, the vast terrain external to human health has become opened to more clinical investigation (Brown 1974; Benson 1975, 1979, Pelletier 1976, 1979, Bresler 1979). Behavioral medicine seeks to encompass the major portion of health services devoted to managing psychological, social, and environmental factors determining patients' health (Carr and Dengerink 1983). Identification of individual risk factors and appropriate preventive interventions are starting to be incorporated. While these efforts are a long overdue expansion of medical practice, they remain primarily focused upon the individual. Because they usually fall short of primary prevention – stopping disease before it actually starts – (Kane 1976), strategies directed at larger social levels are needed to accompany them.

That social conditions largely account for health status in a given population poses the problem of human maladaption to the specific psycho-social and environmental stressors of modern existence – a point concerning many thinkers about health (Eyer and Sterling 1977). What is the wisdom of attempting to adjust individuals to a health-damaging workplace if work alienation results in lower general psychological and physical well-being? (Garfield 1980; Coburn 1983). The occupational health literature is replete with studies revealing more serious health consequences emanating from pathogenic conditions under which people labor (Hamilton and Hardy 1974; Stellman and Daum 1975; Zenz 1975; Kusnetz and Hutchinson 1977; Berman 1978; Navarro and Berman 1983). Numerous incidences of adverse health effects from certain consumer products, toxic waste disposal, nuclear reactor byproducts, and other environmental hazards appear more a matter of news than study. Corporate production needs to circumscribe a wide range of new industrial medicine endeavors based upon behavioral medicine precepts (Greene 1983). The danger lies in management minimizing or masking the workplace origins of exposure and stress-related problems.

In questioning the merits to merely changing personal habits, I do not mean to belittle recent developments in and positive extensions of clinical practice. Research in psychosomatics (Lipowski 1977) holds great promise. Yet, many practitioners promoting "stress management" for individual patients often seem unconcerned about the coincident erosion of the public health tradition, and rarely search out to change larger connections to disease causation. Simply "renewing one's internal environment," as many of the new holistic therapies suggest, is a necessary, but insufficient as well as difficult, option for many folk under social siege beyond their coping.

Health and social conditions in the world

Despite the application of medical science and technology, higher standards of living, and other social and public health advances lessening the distribution of illness, a significant portion of the world's citizenry today remains ill. The brutal fact is that more human beings are sick, suffering, and starving than at any other time in the past. What makes this of special consequence is that for the first time in history the people of the world realize that their poor health and social misery does not need to be their inescapable fate (Stavrianos 1976). From the flow of international information and communication networks that have "shrunk" the world, people know that proper nutrition, pure water, adequate sanitary facilities, and immunizations and antibiotics can greatly reduce their afflictions.

A significant portion of populations in the advanced industrial nations are also ill (Sidel and Sidel 1979). As Dubos indicated, diseases may be eradicated or diminished, but other conditions become prevalent. On one hand, poor health is not an inevitable or unchangeable condition for humanity, but a product of social conditions in each nation of the world. The dramatic transformation of health in the People's Republic of China testifies to this (Horn 1969; Sidel and Sidel 1972; Kleinman *et al.* 1975; Garfield and Salmon 1981). On the other hand, the fact is that people are beset with a ubiquity of potential pathogens – from the microbial, chemical, climatic, radioactive, psychological, social, and cultural. So why not even greater disease?

Antonovsky (1980) has asked this poignant question in a search for what in the very fabric of life, both individually and socially, leads some people to succumb to bombardment from these numerous pathogens, while others remain prone toward health. In studies on stressors related to health, illness, and patienthood, he and his colleagues looked at people's ability to overcome such stressors in terms of "generalized resistance resources." These provide one with a set of meaningful coherent life experiences and enable the employment of various means to get through stress events with lesser degrees of damage. "Salutogenesis," his concept of the ultimate mystery of some host resistance to disease, is an interesting contribution to thinking about health. It is also a useful bridge to cosmological suppositions receiving popular attention recently.

The cosmological connection

Concepts of health have taken on many diverse meanings and values from culture to culture across human history. Just as the social context of health has been forgotten or continues to be unseen, proponents of holism claim that the plan of the whole was lost in modern society. In contrast to the crude materialism of scientific medicine, a common element in preceding alternative systems of medicine is the notion of a "life force."

Sometimes called "Chi," "Ki," "Prana," "vitalism," this life force is said to be integral to health and healing (White and Krippner 1977). Disease is said to be an imbalance (Palos 1972). Rebalancing of body energies remains a cardinal principle of homoeopathy, naturopathy, chiropractic, and acupuncture, besides Feldenkrais, Alexander technique, polarity, shiatsu, and other body massage (Berkeley Holistic Health Center 1978; Kaslof 1979).

There is an implied unity or oneness between the person and nature, a cosmological connection which is said to account for an innate healing potential within the person and from an external universal healing source. Krieger sums up:

> There is a universal meaning or order in the world of the ancients which is reflected in human beings. When the macrocosmic order is undistorted, the microcosm (man/woman) is in a state of well-being. The potentialities of this order are mobilized through a dual interchange of energies [i.e. Yin–Yang] that affects the individual through a non-material, multidimensional network. This net is vitalized by a universal life energy . . . conditioned through the cyclic phenomena of time and becomes apparent as the humors of the body. The combinations of these humors result in the personality characteristics of the individual. Other factors affecting the individual's well-being are climate, seasons of the year, geographic location, the individual's nutritional status, age, sex, and temperament, and the manner in which he or she conducts the daily acts of life.   (Krieger 1981: 127)

The loss of a spiritual dimension in health and healing came with the elevation of science over religion across the last century and a half. When the body became viewed more as a machine with the natural occurrence of disease located in the individual, treatment logically was extended to individualized biomedical intervention to fight disease. Nebulous interactions were relegated to lesser importance, or in most cases, excluded from consideration as non-material.

Due to their feudal, pre-scientific origins, some alternative medicines have focused mainly on the patient's response to illness, not on disease as we now conceive it. Sobel sees the difference as:

Western scientific medicine is largely concerned with the
objective, non-personal, physicochemical explanations of
disease as well as its technical control. In contrast, many
traditional systems of healing are . . . aimed principally at
providing meaningful and understandable explanations of
illness experience.   (Sobel 1979: 108)

The unique response of the person was a theoretical foundation of modern medicine too. It was reflected in the admonition
of Dr William Osler, the famous American medical scientist at
the turn of this century: to treat the patient who has the disease,
not just the disease that the patient has. Adherence to this
construct does not in itself guarantee a consistent medical practice. Conceptually, however, it does allow for a fuller accounting of the incredibly complex and interrelated dynamics of
disease causation, onset, progression, and alleviation, including physiological, psychological, social, cultural, as well as the
spiritual.

Today's resurrection of alternative systems likewise does not
necessarily bring along a recognition of the cultural, social, and
spiritual legacy upon which they were founded. In many cases,
practitioners of alternative therapeutics, like their scientific
counterparts, place greater emphasis on technique, having
modernized and reinterpreted earlier notions. What really
happens in the modern, commodified form of pre-scientific,
traditional medicines is that the social network dimension
disappears as the spiritual dimension is reified. Many contemporary holistic health entrepreneurs 'jump over' the social and
connect the isolated individual to a surrealized metaphysical
universe. Just as the isolated individual is an unrealistic category, so are many interpretations of the spiritual realm. Modern
holistic practitioners are not the only people who do this
tranformation of reality; it has a long tradition in religious
circles.

When any practitioner assigns critical importance to their
interpersonal relations and rituals, the *Gestalt* of the
practitioner–patient relationship takes on new meaning (Frank
1963). A more thorough review of healing would thus require
just as much scrutiny over the interactional field, investigating
procedures, beliefs and notions, non-verbal communication,
meanings of spoken words, and more. With a new interpretation

of past spiritual referents and principles, the study of "morpho-genetic," gravitational, and magnetic fields is now thought to give clues to an "entrapment of spirit in matter," thus pro-viding a new lens to understanding interpersonal healing (Grad 1971–72; Krippner and Villoldo 1976; Meek 1977; de Vries 1981). The qualities of presence, genuineness, empathy, and unconditional positive regard by practitioners have long been identified as presenting a healing force (Cousins 1976, 1977, 1983), though not materially measurable in their fullness as yet.

Modern reviewers of this cosmological notion of oneness see the mind field connecting the person to forces in nature and the universe. Theoretical suppositions about universal laws link healthy human functions, behaviors, and consciousness. Capra (1982) states:

> Because the systems view of mind is not limited to individual organisms but can be extended to social and ecological systems, we may say that groups of people, societies, and cultures have a collective mind, and therefore also possess a collective psyche, which also includes a collective uncon-scious. As individuals we participate in these collective mental patterns, are influenced by them, and shape them in turn. In addition the concepts of planetary mind and a cosmic mind may be associated with planetary and cosmic levels of consciousness.   (Capra 1982: 296)

The age-old aims and disciplines of the sacred traditions offer more than merely expanded theoretical perspective to health. There are downsides to how the spiritual realm is currently being considered. On the one hand, various religious trappings often becloud preciseness in the conceptions. As often applied, the aim is the potentialization of self rather than connected as liberation of human potential within a framework of struggle for social justice and equality toward collective health. On the other hand, powerful uncomprehended spiritual practices (e.g. certain yogic postures, breathing, and meditation techniques) are being clinically employed as a kind of "spiritual technol-ogy." Thought to be therapeutic for all persons to reach "higher levels of consciousness" and to aid in reducing most ills, these pursuits when unsupervised by knowledgeable teachers some-times result in "kundalini accidents," or the clinical damage from the psycho-physiological manifestations of raising of the body's spiritual energy (Gopi Krishna 1975; Sannella 1978; White 1979).

Perhaps in response to the technological rationality and the present mind set of scientific medicine, a significant number of searchers for health, self-actualization, and enlightenment in contemporary society are attracted to the irrational and mystical. This is part of the larger east/west world view clash (Needleman and Lewis 1976; Cox 1979). Along with these cosmological orientations to health and healing comes a critical analysis of the intentions and outcomes of bureaucratic health care institutions and their larger social purposes. Gordon (1984) sees holistic health centers representing attempts to create a locus of care that is not large-scale, insensitive, and technologically cluttered.

The "paradigm shift"

In the early 1970s Thomas Kuhn's argument regarding changes in scientific progress through a series of paradigm shifts (1970) gave impetus to critics of conventional medical care. In a hope to bring together "new" information about culture, ecology, nutrition, exercise and fitness, advocates for a "new medicine" and "new physics" united with parapsychologists in proclaiming a new paradigm with a central focus on "health" – a theme echoed throughout holistic health, consciousness, and spiritual circles, though what is meant varied greatly (O'Regan and Carlson 1979). While physics has often been thought of as the paradigmatic science, not all sciences can be described in such a manner. There are some in which quantification and other mathematic approaches have a high explanatory or heuristic value; functional biology is another. A parallel cannot be drawn for other "sciences," especially most of medicine which has been seen more as a social science (Sigerist 1960). This did not stop advocates of the "paradigm shift" from making the extension, however.

In his book, *The End of Medicine*, Carlson (1975a) saw future cultural developments, including the transformation of consciousness and biological adaptation as the mechanisms for mankind to achieve improved health. The "new medicine" is to draw from the leading edge of psychosomatics, neurophysiology, endocrinology, consciousness research, and a range of alternative therapeutics (White 1974; Carlson 1975b; Pelletier 1979). Its proponents have heralded the "powers of the mind" – newly verifiable abilities to affect what was formerly understood as involuntary functions of the autonomic nervous system (Green 1977; Ehrenwald 1977). These breakthroughs in regulating functions of respiration, digestion, and circulation open up new vistas for both cure and prevention. Moreover, the changes for medicine would rely upon support from what they think is coming in the overall transformation of social institutions (Ferguson 1980).

Various thinkers have been attempting to construct a new conceptual framework for health and human existence. It is acknowledged that some of their formulations and statements are full of supposition and speculation and draw from diverse, not-so-readily-connected perspectives and disciplines. Flynn sums up some philosophical underpinnings to this "paradigm shift:"

> Heisenberg's uncertainty principle, Bell's theorem, the discovery of the brain's own analgesics and the subsequent discovery of many neurotransmitters in the brain, Ilya Prigogine's discovery in chemistry of dissipative structures and change, new insights into the limbic and reticular activating system, research into the hemispheric functions of the brain, biofeedback, self-regulating techniques, and Eastern philosophies and practices are all major events that have led to a paradigm shift. This shift is a revolutionary one which incorporates many new theories, formulae, and hypotheses, describing the function and structure of the world and our presence in it . . . the recent studies of human nature from the fields of anthropology, sociology, biology, and ethology have tended to emphasize the hostile territorial aggressive aspects of human behavior. This pessimistic view needs to be balanced by one which has received little attention: the extraordinary capacity of the human being for loving and caring.   (Flynn 1980: 1)

In this regard, advocates for a whole range of alternative therapeutics have seized upon the "caring versus curing" dichotomy that the nursing profession had earlier proclaimed to differentiate itself from the practice of medicine (George

1980). More personal and intimate relations between practitioner and patient are claimed to recognize and support
the unity and oneness of the universe. The tenet is extracted
from eastern philosophy (Weber 1981). Advocates for holism
in health claim to consider the inseparable connectedness of
the whole universe, the relationship of parts, the processes
within, and interactions and independencies amongst all the
parts.

The critique of scientific medicine by these new paradigm
builders essentially represents an attack on Western thinking:
against reductionism (i.e. knowledge reduced into more simple
ideas); against mechanistic assumptions (i.e. displaying
machine-like qualities which are thus analyzable); and against
atomistic tendencies (i.e. assuming a separate existence of matter and spirit, with only the former able to be elaborated and
understood). Moreover, the dualism of Rene Descartes separating the mind from the body has also been seen as a negative
influence in contemporary medicine. In reducing healing to
mainly therapeutic regimens to alter the physio-chemical
body, due attention has been neglected toward the psychosocial, cultural, ecological, spiritual, and even nutritional
aspects of human health.

Thus, critics of the biomedical model see the need for a major
overhaul of medicine based on a different view of reality. Proposed are new assumptions to enable fuller consideration to and
accounting for the anomalies that scientific medicine has
usually dismissed (for example, the placebo effect and spontaneous remissions). Placing faith in the empirical results
obtained by various alternative therapeutics, the paradigm
builders believe the usual protocols of investigation and publication in standard scientific journals may be too restrictive.
Rather, different ways of researching efficacy to judge how well
the patient responds are suggested, rather than simply measuring the technique or drug. These may reveal why certain alternative therapies seem to work between certain practitioners
and patients. In maintaining that rational and intuitive ways
of knowing are both useful, the paradigm builders question
whether "science" should be conceived of as merely a body of
knowledge sanctioned by an institutional elite. Given the
assumptions of a cosmological connection and interactions
between consciousnesses, research reliability and validity

always remain questionable, as some investigators now claim (Rosenthal 1969; Solfvin 1982).

The "new physics" and health

Proponents of the "new physics" have virtually shaped the contours of discussion regarding the paradigm shift (Capra 1977). What follows is a brief summary of how they conceive the whole universe and whole person to be tied together; and how this unprovable theoretical exposition is said to relate to consciousness and health.

Based on quantum physics, this thinking has attempted to construct a new framework for understanding reality, mind, and the universe. It directly challenges what is felt to be the closed-mindedness in dominant scientific circles, medicine, and general thought. Capra (1982) explains how this modernist view emerged out of twentieth century physical sciences and mathematics after Einstein's influence. It places emphasis on interrelational, indeterminate, and probabilistic qualities to matter and energy. As such, it counters Newtonian determinism, realism, and linear causality – components that underlie the scientific method.

It is important to note that origins of Newtonian physics date back to when western society was changing from a feudal to capitalist form of organization – a point rarely pointed out by these commentators. Coincident development of the western world view, "scientific advancement," and dramatic advances in the productive economic forces have established many linkages. Over this course of time, rationalist conceptions guiding the pursuit of "scientific knowledge" became ever more narrowly derived from the scientific method. In modern society, the scientific method has been held to be a reliable, value-free, and non-political basis upon which to rest judgments. Of course, this has been well contested in many quarters, and the thinkers under discussion offer a totally new lens for initially perceiving phenomena.

The British physicist Bohm sees, as a fundamental aspect of reality, an implicate order to the universe composed of frequencies beyond time and space that has been hidden from us. He maintains that we live in a holographic universe of unending complexity, but not beyond the partial comprehension of humankind. By this he means that all the information of the universe is contained in its parts; there is a cohesive interconnectedness. In the same vein, Stanford neurophysiologist Pribram (1978a) maintains that the deeper structures of the brain are analogous to a hologram, in that they are encoded to produce information about the whole. This is derived from the fact that a surgically removed portion of brain tissue does not destroy memory. As a single gene contains the whole, memory seems distributed throughout the whole brain. The patterned electrical activity of the neurons in Pribram's opinion work holographically.

The holographic model is borrowed from photography. A localized space–time of an ordinary photograph is changed into a holographic representation by passing a laser beam through the film. This yields a different three dimensional perspective (or information) depending on the angle of observation or the way one observes. A small piece of the photographic plate renders the complete picture, that is to say the part contains the information of the whole. Applying this analogously to brain function and ultimately to the universe allows the postulation that relativity inextricably links time and space. The arbitrary divisions of matter and energy; and of past, present, and future can no longer be maintained. This mode of thinking has brought new theoretical insights to quantum mechanics, neurophysiology, and healing.

Pribram (1978b) has said:

> I believe that the paradigm shift in science occasioned by the insights obtained in quantum physics and carried forward by the holographic model of brain function will, in fact, provide us with the base of understanding which makes it clear that the world of appearance is but a reciprocal of another reality, a reality that may already have been explored experientially for untold millennia.   (Pribram 1978b: 87)

The meaning and implications of the holographic suppositions of Pribram and Bohm are extensive; their application to health has been attempted by a few writers. My attempt here is not to explicate or defend this perspective, but to merely note its presence in order for the reader to ponder possible influences on the social definition of health.

Dossey (1983) asks:

> if Bohm's contention is correct, that the entire universe and
> everything in it can only be understood as an inseparable
> entity describable by quantum theory, how can we possibly
> retain our ordinary ideas of what bodies, health, and disease
> actually mean? Human bodies, spacially separated, seem to
> be noncausally and nonlocally inseparable in a modern
> physical view; and health and disease, as collected moments
> in time, also take on a noncausal and nonlocal oneness . . .
> Our habitual way of describing isolated healthy bodies as
> being recurrently besieged by spells of poor health from birth
> to the grave has to be reevaluated in any modern description
> of the world. If moments in time are inseparable, then so are
> health and disease. If elements in space are inseparable, then
> so are our bodies. And if time and space are inseparable, then
> our bodies are one with the health and disease that we tradi-
> tionally presume they "possess" in some alternating
> sequence.   (Dossey 1983: 111)

Basically, these thinkers see the body with a certain individuality, but it is highly dependent on the environment to exist
(Bohm 1980). External factors affect health at the level of
"frequencies" (Ferguson 1978a). The body is more clearly
attuned to the "primary level of reality" where the holographic
explanation of the interactions of fields are "in phase" for
health generating, while "out-of-phase experience" leads to
"disrhythmias." There are thus complex, multiple causations
to illness or wellness depending on the integrity of impacting
energy fields. Breaks in harmony lead to disease states. The
mind results from previous interactions with the environment,
but also reflects the basic organization of the universe (Pribram
1976). The mind and the body are intrinsically united, and
consciousness is the fulcrum of health (Dossey 1983: 189). As
there are "holomovements" in the universe, so the individual's consciousness toward a spiritual reality reflects such a
dynamic in which all living entities are interconnected in an
"ocean of energy" (Bohm 1978). Thus health and disease are
primarily attributed to consciousness, not the gross physical
field (Weber 1981). Ferguson (1978b) maintains that self-
responsibility for positive wellness is important for self-
healing, which comes with "resonance" of energies, and is
obtained from the design of one's consciousness. Its outward

manifestations – psychological factors, emotions, feelings – are receptive to significant modification in altered states (meditation, biofeedback, hypnosis, imagery, and visualization, and like "mind" therapies).

Benor (1983) notes:

> This apparent duality within the brain, including diffuse and discrete modes of function, seems to parallel aspects of man's perceptions of the world which have puzzled religious luminaries, philosophers, and scientists throughout the ages. Man, experiencing the world through his five everyday senses, perceives himself as discrete from other persons and objects around him. Yet on other levels, such as in meditation, he perceives himself as one with the universe. The apparent contradiction between these various perceptions must be due to the differences in the various modalities available to man for experiencing the world.
>
> (Benor 1983: 107)

Noting the holographic premise that the part contains the whole, Benor mentions that the foot, hand, ear, eye, and other parts of the body have been claimed to correlate aspects of personality, emotional states, health, and disease. Reich and his bioenergetic followers maintain that body structure also correlates with one's intrapsychic nature (Reich 1961; Lowen 1971, 1975). Such assumptions are common among various holistic-styled practitioners.

Premises derived from this thinking are claimed to aid explanations of psychic or spiritual healing (Benor 1984) as well as various psychic states (for example, clairvoyance, telepathy, precognition, etc.) (O'Regan 1981). Transpersonal "resonance" between the energy fields of a healer and healee provides for effectiveness from the interaction, and it supposedly has even greater effects. Dossey maintains: "Health is not just an individual affair. Like disease, it can be spread. Efforts toward health care, therefore, transcend the actions of single individuals. What one person does to improve – or to diminish – his health has vital consequences to all other persons" (Dossey 1983: 143).

According to this viewpoint, health creating activities affect the affairs of the entire human race. Thus, the supposition of world-changing implications leads some followers of this orientation to leap to social change perspectives of an *Aquarian Conspiracy*, a *Third Wave* and *Turning Point* in history of the coming New Age (Ferguson 1980; Toffler 1981; Capra 1982).

The development of this whole line of argument regarding the paradigm shift is only beginning to be elaborated. At yet it is not sufficiently detailed, being more acceptable to and contemplated by those hopeful for significant social transformation. It certainly has not captured the interests of medical scientists, nor mainstream thought. Disregarding problems with its substance, the unconventional character of this reasoning – its appeal to higher qualities of humankind and to the supernatural – seem to make it attractive to a particular variety of searcher today. The number of conferences offered and books sold on eastern philosophy and religion, parapsychology and the occult, and holistic health care indicates a rather large audience for this kind of orientation to health. Unlike Galileo though, many of these New Age vocalists personally and materially gain from their pronouncements and positions.

There is little reason at this time to believe the above described thinking will significantly influence dominant social thought. This spiritual–physical conception of human consciousness suggests a re-evaluation (and a discarding) of many key notions about health under scientific medicine. The integrative attempts of the "new paradigm" to aid explanatory capabilities over anomalies in health and consciousness await more theoretical and model development, in addition to substance. In general, these speculations, especially as they posit the universe operating on different, even volitionally arbitrary principles, clearly parallel the surrealized, reified spiritual sphere to which alternative medicine advocates constantly appeal for ultimate healing energy. Though imaginative and dramatic, these physical speculations and suppositions often represent once again the attempt of thinkers out of the mainstream to find followings for their intellectual ponderings out of the disaffection within the literate middle-class populace.

Yet a philosophical point of interest arises out of the proclaimed science and religion compatibility. Being less concerned with validity in their conceptualizations, I find the orientation and methodology may contribute to discussions about health and may eventually lead to an upgrading of critiques of alternative systems of medicine. Implied is a search for values through reflection upon both one's inner struggle for meaning and the cultural potentials. Hopefully, the sense of an ecological system of consciousness will link adherents in alliance with groups struggling against concrete social and environmental pathogenesis. This of course depends upon the extent that cosmological or spiritual extractions from these theoretical ponderings related to health and healing give practitioners and clients a greater commitment to work toward a more collective health.

Political economic developments in health care

Knowledge is a social product dependent on the social activity of real world actors. It is not just intellectual discourse. A case here is "medical science," which has flourished to such a degree only with strong social institutional support. Today dissatisfactions with some notions and conceptions of scientific medicine have become widespread, extending from popular to powerful circles. Once revered for its paradigms and institutions, it now reveals to some an incompleteness. A growing, restless social constituency appears ready to move on to updated and revitalized perspectives on health and healing. We are in the midst of a transition period of conflicting ideas, ideologies, paradigms, and theories that need much sorting out. Whatever course these wanderings may take, people will do so under concrete social conditions. The changing institutional context of health care delivery thus bears examination.

The health care sector of the US economy has been increasingly concentrating, away from its previous small-scale, generally "not-for-profit" orientation. Over the next two decades nationwide health care corporations will become providers of health services to a major portion of the American population (Salmon 1984). Rapidly growing across the 1970s, these large-scale corporate entities have been seeking international markets; six US hospital management firms own or operate over twenty hospitals in Great Britain (Federation of American Hospitals, 1982).

The editor of *The New England Journal of Medicine* sees this "new medical industrial complex" as the "most important recent development in American health care" (Relman 1981: 963). Firms such as Hospital Corporation of America, American Medical International, Humana, National Medical Enterprises,

Charter Medical Corporations, among about twenty other proprietary hospital chains, have been expanding beyond hospital
services. Many are diversifying into nursing home, hemo-
dialysis, diagnostic lab, ambulatory care, home care, hospital
contract management, and a variety of other services. While
the total number of hospitals in the US has been declining,
the investor-owned hospital segment has increased; now they
own 15 per cent of non-government acute general beds (and
more than half of non-government psychiatric beds). Estimates
range between 25–30 per cent for their ownership by the end of
the decade, not including the large number of "not-for-profit"
institutions under management contract with the corporate
hospital chains. Besides these chains, several commercial
insurance companies and multi-state health maintenance
organizations (e.g. Cigma, Prudential, John Hancock, Kaiser-
Permanente) are moving to begin large-scale ambulatory care
operations across the country. This proprietarization thrust
has been gaining legitimacy by appealing to the cost efficiency
demands of the federal goverment and large corporate employers
who purchase medical care benefits for their workers (Salmon 1980).

Also during the 1970s was an unprecedented involvement of
these large corporate "purchasers" in health policy and
planning and in the direct provision of health services for their
employees. Corporate planning and lobbying bodies, such as
the Washington Business Group on Health, the Conference
Board, the National Chamber Foundation, Interstudy of
Minneapolis, Boston University's Center for Industry and
Health Care, among others, began actions to reorganize the
health care delivery system (Salmon 1977). In numerous locations around the US, corporations began integrating family and
industrial medicine at the workplace; initiating preventive
medicine, health education, and fitness and wellness programs;
rearranging employee health benefit packages; sponsoring and
backing health maintenance organizations and other new
delivery forms; and setting up local business coalitions to
monitor health provider behavior (Salmon 1978). These actions
arose out of the need to stem increases in health expenses and to
improve worker productivity, and thus corporate returns on
investment. The policies and pursuits of these powerful agents
of social and economic development must be accorded great

significance, not only in the discussions on the social definition of health, but also in the reorganizing of medicine.

The interstices of the new thinking on health with these two developments should be apparent. Re-designing medical activity into highly-centralized nationwide firms will assuage corporate class entities who seek rationalization of a chaotic, costly, and inefficient delivery system. Thus, health care by the end of this decade will be transformed to be more "business-like" and "efficient." With their predominant purpose being profit, proprietary provider organizations appear willing to adapt to "consumer demands" for a broader "health product." Already, numerous holistic health entrepreneurs have begun peddling their "new, improved" wares to corporate clients willing to buy. Related policy discussions are thus important to the interests of all these parties to develop strategies for greater legitimation of health care under capitalism (Salmon and Berliner 1980).

This author is not so ready to foresee a total eclipse of scientific medicine – either from the garnering of age-old wisdom from past alternative medicines, or from these new speculations on health, healing, and human existence. It would be naive to predict scientific medicine even ending its disease focus in the near future; its orientation is institutionally well embedded. The beginning societal responses in health promotion and prevention under corporate auspices are however extending the province of health care institutional activity, and coincidentally lessening medical authority. There are many more implications of the forthcoming industrialization by nationwide provider systems that bear upon the changing content of health and medical services.

Predicting specific outcomes here would be just as speculative as some of the above thinking about health. However, one final point is relevant to the discussion of health. In modern society, all services, products, and even information to create "health" has been reduced to a commodity transaction between a buyer and a seller. This is inimical to the human need for health to be enjoyed, not consumed. Trends toward corporate patenting of bio-technology, advanced surgical techniques and procedures, and human "spare" parts further portend a contradictory economic orientation. The "bottom line" consideration of profit in health care may, and often does, compromise quality, effectiveness, and value. Profit potentials also dictate the nature and kind of service provided in our society and to whom. Where human beings themselves are viewed as commodities, individuals become valued differently by their contribution to economic production. This destroys inner spiritual purpose and the aim of work to achieve social meaningfulness, in addition to separating us from the experience of our collective health.

Conclusion

This chapter has presented a range of ideas concerning what constitutes human health and preconditions necessary for its enhancement. I have attempted to demonstrate the political importance to the social definition of health, maintaining that the character of the entire institutional development in health care may flow from it. The material and ideological conditions of modern society provide for complex interpenetrations to the issue. Variations on defining health described here bear watching to more fully assess their elaboration and respective influence over time.

Today the diversity and ambiguity in the idea of health has provided for an even greater variety of meanings assigned to its experience by people. The current popular interest is too vast to characterize precisely and entirely, but it continues to be influenced by cultural and political economic aspects noted in the above discussion. The importance to how the social definition of health evolves over the next few decades extends beyond boundaries of philosophical discourse; it will ideologically circumscribe elements of health policy and the reorganizing of medicine.

Resolutions to the multi-faceted problems of health and health care are being pursued within the present political economic and cultural framework. The apparent course provides for little democratic determination over health care institutions in order to serve more fully the broader health needs in the entire population. It is likely that the "new medical industrial complex" of nationwide providers will, over time, exploit popular sentiments for a broader range of services, but only for those in the population able to pay. Nevertheless, organized health care corporations will be unable to overcome the social production of disease inherent in an economy which in so many ways places profit considerations above human needs. Nor will these large-scale firms probably employ means to promote healing based upon deeper dimensions of human existence, though renditions on packaging holistic-styled services can be expected if a "market" for such promises handsome returns on investment.

People experience more to the nature of health than the commodified "product" of profit-based health care can ever provide. Therefore, these political economic directions will be continually resisted through personal and popular struggle for the construction of a more healthy society and ecology, within which the practice of healing disease and illnesses can be structurally assisted. In my opinion, achieving a consensus on broadening and clarifying the concept of health is vital for political opposition to corporate and government erosion of health protection for workers, consumers, and our social and ecological environment (Navarro 1982).

References

Aaron, H.J. and Schwartz, W.B. (1984) *The Painful Prescription: Rationing Hospital Care*. Washington, DC: Brookings Institution.

Ackerknecht, E.H. (1953) *Rudolf Virchow: Doctor, Statesman, Anthropologist*. Madison, WI: University of Wisconsin Press.

——(1968) *A Short History of Medicine*. New York: The Ronald Press.

Albright, P. and Albright, B.P. (eds) (1980) *Body, Mind and Spirit*. Brattleboro, Vermont: The Stephen Greene Press.

Antonovsky, A. (1980) *Health, Stress, and Coping*. San Francisco: Jossey-Bass.

Ardell, D.B. (1977) *High Level Wellness*. Emmaus, Pa: Rodale Press.

Benor, D.J. (1983) Intersections of Holography, Psi, Acupuncture, and Related Issues. *American Journal of Acupuncture* 11(2): 105–18.

——(1984) Psychic Healing. In J. Warren Salmon (ed.) *Alternative Medicines: Popular and Policy Perspectives*. New York: Methuen. London: Tavistock.

Benson, H. (1975) *The Relaxation Response*. New York: William Morrow.

282   *Alternative medicines*

——(1979) *The Mind/Body Effect*. New York: Simon & Schuster.

Berkeley Holistic Health Center (1978) *The Holistic Health Handbook*. Berkeley: And/Or Press.

Berkman, L.F. and Syme, S.L. (1979) Social Networks, Host Resistance and Mortality. *American Journal of Epidemiology* 109: 186–204.

Berliner, H.S. (1983) Medical Modes of Production. In P. Wright and A. Treacher (eds) *The Social Construction of Medicine*. Edinburgh: University of Edinburgh Press.

Berliner, H.S. and Salmon, J.W. (1979) The New Realities of Health Policy and Influence of Holistic Medicine. *Journal of Alternative Human Services* 5(2): 13–16.

Berliner, H.S. and Salmon, J.W. (1980) The Holistic Alternative to Scientific Medicine: History and Analysis. *International Journal of Health Services* 10(1): 133–47.

Berman, D.M. (1978) *Health on the Job*. New York: Monthly Review Press.

Bohm, D. (1978) The Enfolding-Unfolding Universe. *ReVision* 1(3/4): 24–51.

——(1980) *Wholeness and The Implicate Order*. London: Routledge & Kegan Paul.

Bohm, D. and Weber, R. (1983) Of Matter and Meaning: The Super-Implicate Order. *ReVision* 6(1): 34–44.

Braverman, H. (1974) *Labor and Monopoly Capital*. New York: Monthly Review Press.

Brenner, H. (1973) *Mental Illness and the Economy*. Cambridge: Harvard University Press.

Bresler, D.E. (1979) *Free Yourself from Pain*. New York: Simon & Schuster.

Brown, B. (1974) *New Mind, New Body*. New York: Harper & Row.

Capra, F. (1977) *The Tao of Physics*. New York: Bantam Books.

——(1982) *The Turning Point: Science, Society, and the Rising Culture*. New York: Bantam Books.

Carlson, R.J. (1975a) *The End of Medicine*. New York: John Wiley.

——(ed.) (1975b) *The Frontiers of Science and Medicine*. Chicago: Henry Regnery.

Carr, J.E. and Dengerink, H.A. (eds) (1983) *Behavioral Science in the Practice of Medicine*. New York: Elsevier.

Coburn, D. (1983) Job Alienation and Well-Being. In V. Navarro and D.M. Berman *Health and Work Under Capitalism*. Farmingdale, New York: Baywood.

Cousins, N. (1976) Anatomy of an Illness. *New England Journal of Medicine* 295: 1458–463.

——(1977) The Mysterious Placebo: How the Mind Helps Medicine

Work. *Saturday Review* 1 October: 8–12.

——(1983) *The Healing Heart*. New York: W.V. Norton.

Cox, H. (1979) *Turning East: The Promise and Peril of the New Orientalism*. New York: Touchstone.

Crawford, R. (1977) You Are Dangerous to your Health: The Ideology and Politics of Victim Blaming. *International Journal of Health Services* 7(4): 663–80.

Dossey, L. (1983) *Space, Time, And Medicine*. Boulder: Shambala.

Dreitzel, H.P. (1971) *The Social Organization of Health*. New York: Macmillan.

Dubos, R. (1965) *Man Adapting*. New Haven, CT: Yale University Press.

——(1968) *Man, Medicine and Environment*. New York: Frederick A. Praeger.

Ehrenwald, J. (1977) Psi Phenomena and Brain Research. In B. Wolman *Handbook of Parapsychology*. New York: Van Nostrand Rheinhold.

Engel, G. (1977) The Need for a New Medical Model: A Challenge for Biomedicine. *Science* 196: 129–36.

Estes, C.L. (1979) *The Aging Enterprise*. San Francisco: Jossey-Bass.

——(1982) Austerity and Aging in the US: 1980 and Beyond. *International Journal of Health Services* 12(4): 573–84.

Evans, R.W. (1983) Health Care Technology and the Inevitability of Resource Allocation and Rationing Decisions. *Journal of the American Medical Association*. Pt I, 249(15): 2047–053; Pt II, 249(16): 2208–222.

Eyer, J. (1977) Prosperity as a Cause of Death. *International Journal of Health Services*. 7(1): 125–50.

——(1984) Capitalism, Health and Illness. In J.B. McKinlay *Issues in the Political Economy of Medical Care*. New York: Methuen. London: Tavistock Publications.

Eyer, J. and Sterling, P. (1977) Stress-related Mortality and Social Organization. *Review of Radical Political Economics* 9: 1–44.

Federation of American Hospitals (1982) *The 1983 Directory: Investor-owned Hospitals and Hospital Management Companies*. Little Rock, Ark: Federation of American Hospitals.

Ferguson, M. (1980) *The Aquarian Conspiracy: Personal and Social Transformation in the 1980s*. New York: St Martin.

——(1978a) Karl Pribram's Changing Reality. *ReVision* 1(3/4) 8–13.

——(1978b) A New Perspective on Reality. *Mind/Brain Bulletin* 3: 1–4.

Flynn, P.A.R. (1980) *Holistic Health: The Art and Science of Care*. Bowie, MD: Robert Brady.

Frank, J. (1963) *Persuasion and Healing: A Comparative Study of Psychotherapy*. New York: Schocken.

Fry, S.T. (1983) Rationing Health Care: The Ethics of Cost Containment. *Nursing Economics* 1: 165–69.

Galdston, I. (1952) *The Meaning of Social Medicine*. Cambridge: Harvard University Press.

Garfield, J. (1980) Alienated Labor, Stress, and Coronary Disease. *International Journal of Health Services* 10(4): 551–61.

Garfield, R. and Salmon, J.W. (1981) Struggles over Health Care in the People's Republic of China. *Journal of Contemporary Asia*. 11: 91–103.

George, J.B. (1980) *Nursing Theories: The Base for Professional Nursing Practice*. Englewood Cliffs, NJ: Prentice-Hall.

Goldbeck, W.B. (1978) *A Business Perspective on Industry and Health Care*. New York: Springer-Verlag.

Gopi Krishna (1975) *The Awakening of the Kundalini*. New York: E.P. Dutton.

Gordon, J. (1984) Holistic Health Centers in the US. In J.W. Salmon (ed.) *Alternative Medicines: Popular and Policy Perspectives*. New York: Methuen. London: Tavistock Publications.

Grad, B. (1971–72) Some Biological Effects of "Laying on of Hands." *Journal of Pastoral Counseling* 6: 38–42.

Green, E. and Green, A. (1977) *Beyond Biofeedback*. New York: Delta.

Greene, J. (1983) Detecting the Hypersusceptible Worker: Genetics and Politics in Industrial Medicine. *International Journal of Health Services*. 13(2): 247–64.

Hamilton, A. and Hardy, H. (1974) *Industrial Toxicology*. Acton, MA: Publishing Sciences Group.

Hastings, A.C., Fadiman, J., and Gordon, J.S. (1980) *Health for the Whole Person*. Boulder, Colorado: Westview Press.

Horn, J.S. (1969) *"Away With All Pests . . .": An English Surgeon in People's China*. New York: Monthly Review Press.

Illich, I. (1976) *Medical Nemesis*. New York: Pantheon.

Kane, R.L. (1976) Disease Control: What is Really Preventable? In *The Challenge of Community Medicine*. New York: Springer.

Kaslof, L.J. (1979) *Wholistic Dimensions in Healing*. New York: Doubleday.

Kelman, S. (1975) The Social Nature of the Definition Problem in Health. *International Journal of Health Services*. 5(4): 626–42.

Kleinman, A., Kunstadter, P., Alexander, E.R., and Gale, J.L. (1975) *Medicine in Chinese Cultures*. Washington, DC: US Govt Printing Office.

Knowles, J. (1976) *Doing Better, Feeling Worse*. New York: W.W. Norton.

Krieger, D. (1981) *Foundations for Holistic Health Nursing Practices: The Renaissance Nurse*. Philadelphia: J.B. Lippincott.

Krippner, S. and Villoldo, A. (1976) *The Realms of Healing*. Millbrae, CA: Celestial Arts.

Kuhn, T.S. (1962) *The Structure of Scientific Revolutions*. Chicago: University of Chicago Press.

Kusnetz, S. and Hutchinson, M. (1977) *Occupational Diseases – A Guide to their Recognition*. (Department of HEW, DHEW Publication No. 79–116; GPO Stock No. 017–033–00266–5). Washington, DC: US Govt Printing Office.

LaPatra, J. (1978) *Healing*. New York: McGraw-Hill.

Lasch, C. (1978) *The Culture of Narcissism*. New York: Norton.

Lipowski, Z.J. (1977) Psychosomatic Medicine in the Seventies: An Overview. *American Journal of Psychiatry*. 134(3): 233–44.

Lowen, A. (1971) *The Language of the Body*. New York: Macmillan.

——(1975) *Bioenergetics*. New York: Penguin.

Maslow, A. (1962) *Toward a Psychology of Being*. Princeton, NJ: Van Nostrand.

McKinlay, J.B. (ed.) (1984) *Issues in the Political Economy of Medical Care*. New York: Methuen. London: Tavistock Publications.

Mechanic, D. (1978) Rationing Medical Care. *The Center Magazine*. September–October: 22–5.

——(1979) *Future Issues in Health Care: Social Policy and the Rationing Medical Services*. New York: The Free Press.

Meek, G. (ed.) (1977) *Healers and the Healing Process*. Wheaton, Ill.: Theosophical Publishing House.

Minkler, M. (1983) Blaming the Aged Victim: The Politics of Scapegoating in Times of Fiscal Conservatism. *International Journal of Health Services* 13(1): 155–68.

Moser, R.H. (1980) The Scientific Marketplace and the Medical Establishment. *Western Journal of Medicine* 132: 160–61.

Naisbett, J. (1982) *Megatrends*. New York: Warner Books.

Navarro, V. (1976) *Medicine Under Capitalism*. New York: Prodist.

——(1982) Where is the Popular Mandate? *New England Journal of Medicine* 307(24): 1516–517.

Navarro, V. and Berman, D. (1983) *Health and Work Under Capitalism*. New York: Baywood Publishing Co.

Needleman, J. and Lewis, D. (1976) *On the Way to Self-Knowledge*. New York: Alfred A. Knopf.

O'Regan, B. (ed.) (1981) Landscapes of the Mind: Perspective on Consciousness Research from Past and Present. *Institute of Noetic Sciences Newletter*. 9(2): 1, 12.

O'Regan, B. and Carlson, R. (1979) Defining Health: The State of the Art. *Holistic Health Review*. 3: 86–101.

Otto, H.A. and Knight, J.W. (eds) (1979) *Dimensions in Wholistic Healing*. Chicago: Nelson-Hall.

Palos, S. (1972) *The Chinese Art of Healing*. New York: Bantam Books.

Parsons, T. (1972) The Sick Role and the Role of the Physician Reconsidered. *Milbank Memorial Foundation Quarterly* 53(3): 257–78.

Pelletier, K.R. (1976) *Mind as Healer, Mind as Slayer*. New York: Delta/Delacorte.

——(1979) *Holistic Medicine: From Stress to Optimum Health*. New York: Delcorte Press.

Powles, J. (1973) On the Limitations of Modern Medicine. *Science, Medicine and Man*. 1: 1–30.

Pribram, K.H. (1976) Problems Concerning the Structure of Consciousness. In G. Globus (ed.) *Consciousness and the Brain*. New York: Plenum Press.

——(1978a) A Progress Report on the Scientific Understanding of Paranormal Phenomena. *Proceedings of the International Conference, Montreal*. New York: Parapsychological Foundation.

——(1978b) What the Fuss Is All About. *ReVision*. Summer/Fall: 14–19.

Reich, W. (1961) *Character Analysis*. New York: Farrar, Straus & Giroux.

Relman, A.S. (1981) The New Medical Industrial Complex. *The New England Journal of Medicine*. 303: 963–70.

Renaud, M. (1975) On the Structural Constraints to State Intervention in Health. *International Journal of Health Services* 5(4): 559–72.

Rosen, G. (1958) *A History of Public Health*. New York: MD Publications.

Rosenthal, R. (1969) Interpersonal Expectations: Effects of the Experimenter's Hypothesis. In R. Rosenthal and R.L. Rosnow (eds) *Artifact in Behavioral Research*. New York: Academic Press.

Salmon, J.W. (1975) The Health Maintenance Organization Strategy: A Corporate Takeover of Health Services Delivery. *International Journal of Health Services* 5(4): 609–29.

——(1977) Monopoly Capital and the Reorganization of Health Care. *Review of Radical Political Economics* 9(12): 125–33.

——(1978) *Corporate Attempts to Reorganize the American Health Care System*. Unpublished dissertation, Cornell University.

——(1982) The Competitive Health Strategy: Fighting for Your Health. *Health and Medicine* 1(2): 21–30.

——(1984) Organizing Medical Care for Profit. In J. McKinlay (ed.) *Issues in the Political Economy of Health Care*. New York: Methuen. London: Tavistock Publications.

Salmon, J.W. and Berliner, H.S. (1980) Health Policy Implications of the Holistic Health Movement. *Journal of Health Politics, Policy and Law* 5(3): 535–53.

Sannella, L. (1978) *Kundalini-Psychosis or Transcendence?* San Francisco: H.S. Dakin.

Sidel, V. and Sidel, R. (1972) *Serve the People*. New York: Josiah Macy Foundation.

Sidel, V. and Sidel, R. (1979) *A Healthy State*. New York: Pantheon.

Sigerist, H.E. (1960) The Social History of Medicine. In F. Marti-Ibanez *Henry E. Sigerist On the History of Medicine*. New York: MD Publications.

Simonton, O.C. and Matthews-Simonton, S. (1978) *Getting Well Again*. Los Angeles: J.P. Tarcher.

Smith, J.A. (1981) The Idea of Health: A Philosophic Inquiry. *Advances in Nursing Science* 3(3): 43–50.

Smuts, J.C. (1926) *Holism and Evolution*. New York: Macmillan.

Sobel, D.S. (1979) *Ways of Health*. New York: Harcourt Brace Jovanovich.

Solfvin, G.F. (1982) Psi Expectancy Effect in Psychic Healing Studies with Malarial Mice. *Journal of Parapsychology* 4: 160–97.

Sontag, S. (1977) *Illness as a Metaphor*. New York: Random House.

Stavrianos, L.S. (1976) *The Promise of the Coming Dark Age*. San Francisco: W.H. Freeman.

Stellman, J. and Daum, S. (1975) *Work is Dangerous to Your Health*. New York: Vintage.

Susser, M.W. and Watson, W. (1971) *Sociology in Medicine*. London: Oxford University Press.

Toffler, A. (1981) *The Third Wave*. New York: Bantam Books.

Totman, R. (1979) *Social Causes of Illness*. New York: Pantheon.

Toulmin, S. (1975) Concepts of Function and Mechanism in Medicine and Medical Science. In H. Engelhardt and S. Spicker (eds) *Evaluation and Explanation in the Biosciences*. Boston: D. Reidel.

Travis, J. (1977) *Wellness Inventory*. Mill Valley, CA: Wellness Center.

US Department of Health, Education and Welfare. (1976) *Forward Plan for Health – 1977–1981*. Washington, DC: US Govt Printing Office.

——(1979) *Healthy People: The Surgeon General's Report on Health Promotion and Disease Prevention*. Washington, DC: US Govt Printing Office.

de Vries, (1981) *The Redemption of the Intangible in Medicine*. Rotterdam, Holland: Psychosynthesis Monographs.

Waitzkin, H. (1978) A Marxist View of Medical Care. *Annals of Internal Medicine*. 89: 264–78.

Waldron, I. and Eyer, J. (1975) Socioeconomic Causes of the Recent Rise in Death Rates for 15–24 Year Olds. *Social Science and Medicine* 9: 383–96.

Wartofsky, M. (1975) Organs, Organisms and Disease: Human Ontology and Medical Practice. In H.T. Engelhardt, Jr and S. Spicker *Evaluation and Explanation in the Biomedical Sciences* Boston: D. Reidel.

Weber, R. (1979) Philosophical Foundations and Frameworks for

Healing. *ReVision* 2(3/4): 66–76.

——(1981) Philosophical Foundations and Frameworks for Healing. In M.D. Borelli and P. Heidt (eds) *Therapeutic Touch: A Handbook of Readings*. New York: Springer.

White, J. (1974) *Psychic Exploration: A Challenge for Science*. New York: Paragon Books.

——(1979) *Kundalini, Evolution and Enlightenment*. Garden City, NJ: Anchor Press.

White, J. and Krippner, S. (1977) *Future Science: Life Energies and the Physics of Paranormal Phenomena*. Garden City, NJ: Anchor/Doubleday.

Wright, P. and Treacher, A. (eds) (1983) *The Problem of Medical Knowledge: Examining the Social Construction of Medicine*. Edinburgh: University of Edinburgh Press.

Zenz, C. (1975) *Occupational Medicine: Principles and Practical Applications*. Chicago: Yearbook Medical Publishers.

Acknowledgement

My personal thanks to Doctors Howard S. Berliner, Daniel J. Benor, and Joseph Eyer for comments on a previous draft. Also Agatha M. Gallo provided invaluable assistance and support.

Name index

Subject index